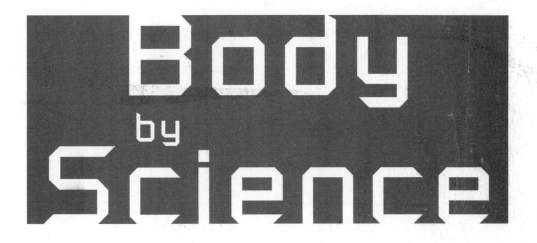

Body by Science

A RESEARCH-BASED PROGRAM FOR STRENGTH TRAINING, BODY BUILDING, AND COMPLETE FITNESS IN 12 MINUTES A WEEK

DOUG McGUFF, M.D., AND JOHN LITTLE

Mc
Graw
Hill

New York Chicago San Francisco Lisbon London Madrid Mexico City
Milan New Delhi San Juan Seoul Singapore Sydney Toronto

Library of Congress Cataloging-in-Publication Data

McGuff, Doug.
  Body by science : a research-based program for strength training, body building,
and complete fitness in 12 minutes a week / Doug McGuff, John Little.
      p.   cm.
  Includes index.
  ISBN 978-0-07-159717-3 (alk. paper)
  1. Exercise.   2. Physical fitness.   3. Weight loss.   4. Bodybuilding—
Physiological aspects.   I. Little, John R., 1960–   II. Title.

GV481.M3975   2009
612'.044—dc22   2008024218

9 10 11 12 13 14 15 16 17 18 19 20 21   DOC/DOC   1 5 4 3 2

ISBN   978-0-07-159717-3
MHID   0-07-159717-4

Interior design by Think Design LLC

McGraw-Hill books are available at special quantity discounts to use as premiums and
sales promotions or for use in corporate training programs. To contact a representative,
please visit the Contact Us pages at www.mhprofessional.com.

This book is printed on acid-free paper.

This book is dedicated to my wife, Wendy; my son, Eric; and my daughter, Madeline. You are my inspiration to be strong and to live as long as possible.

—Doug McGuff, M.D.

To my wife, Terri; to our daughter, Taylor; and to our sons, Riley, Brandon, and Benjamin, who have made me realize just how precious the commodity of time is and why within the family (as opposed to the gym) is the most rewarding place to spend it. This book is also dedicated to a new breed of trainee, who not only truly values his or her time but also demands reasons to justify any impingement of it— particularly while in the pursuit of activities as important as the enhancement of fitness and the maintenance of health.

—John Little

Contents

Acknowledgments

Special thanks go out to my coauthor, John Little. I am honored that you brought me in on this project, and I am grateful for all of your work translating our phone conversations into a treatise on physical training. To Ken Hutchins, thanks for devising the first protocol that raises intensity while lowering force. Thanks also to the late Mike Mentzer, who provided a hero in a time without heroes, and to Terry Carter, who pioneered "time under load" and once-a-week training during the early days of Ultimate Exercise. To the late Clay Brunson, thanks for bringing so much passion and a willingness to experiment to Ultimate Exercise. To Greg Anderson, owner of Ideal Exercise, in Seattle: your insights during hours of discussion helped to shape this book. To Drew Baye and Dr. Ellington Darden, thanks for your excellent websites and writings. To Ryan Hall, thanks for showing us the genetic reasons that one size does not fit all. To Bo Railey, thanks for your business advice and for putting on excellent seminars. To Ed Garbe, my manager at Ultimate Exercise, and instructor Sarah Cooper, thanks for your boundless energy and for keeping it all running. Finally, thank you, Arthur Jones: the man who started it all and whose writings set the course for my life.

—*Doug McGuff, M.D.*

There are many people whom I would like to add to Doug's list. First in order would be Doug McGuff: your insights into global metabolic conditioning and the dose-response relationship of exercise are a work of genius and have advanced people's understanding of the actual science of exercise immeasurably. I also acknowledge the contributions of our medical illustrator, Tim Fedak, whose excellent renderings have allowed for a deeper understanding of muscular function and human metabolism and Gus Diamantopoulos for his charts and diagrams on the nature of the inroading process. In addition, I must acknowledge all of the unheralded personal trainers who have been diligently applying their craft, keeping records, and seeking cause-and-effect relationships for decades. They include expert trainers such as Fred Hahn, Ann Marie Anderson, Doug Holland, David Landau, Terri Little, Cary Howe, Blair Wilson, Chris Greenfield, Daniel Craig, David Wilson, and Jeremy Hymers, who, along with the names Doug cited, represent the absolute top tier of personal trainers on the planet. I would also underscore Doug's acknowledgment of my late friend Mike Mentzer and point out that it was Mike who was the first to thoroughly examine the benefits and necessity of issues such as reduced training volume and frequency on a large-scale basis and who drew many meaningful conclusions from his research that have deepened our understanding of the science of exercise.

—John Little

Introduction

Whom Can You Trust?

How does an average person sift through today's information overload of opinions on health, fitness, and exercise to find factual data in the pursuit of valid knowledge? After all, these fields are rife with varied sources of professed authority, folklore, and even outright deception. How do you know who can be trusted?

THE PROBLEM WITH TESTIMONIALS

The most common mistake that people make in this regard is believing other people. For instance, a testimonial—whether it comes to you from a friend or blares out at you from a TV screen—is a poor criterion for determining truth.

A case in point is the experience of a writer for a popular fitness magazine who once wrote a facetious article about a "miracle supplement." At the bottom of the page on which the article appeared, he had the magazine's art department create a perforated square roughly the size of a postage stamp, next to which appeared the following recommendation: "For optimal muscle gains, cut out this little piece of paper and place it in a glass of water overnight. It contains a special mix of amino acids that are released in water over several hours. In the morning, remove the paper and place it on your tongue to allow the amino acids to enter your body." He intended it as a joke, a last-minute bit of whimsy to fill a page where an advertisement had been withdrawn. His intention, however, was not communicated very well to the readers, as, within days of the magazine's hitting the stands, the publisher was inundated with requests for "more of that awesome paper."

Many readers honestly believed that placing it on their tongues as instructed made their muscles bigger and stronger. This response is characteristic of the placebo effect, a demonstration of the power of suggestion, which impels people to buy all manner of things. If one of your friends or relatives happened to number among those who believed in this "miracle supplement," he or she likely would have told you how "great" this product was, and you—if you put stock in testimonials—would probably have tried it.

While that case was an inadvertent hoax, the credibility of testimonials that appear in advertisements—whether for arthritis-curing bracelets or weight-loss products—is suspect for many reasons. For example, many before-and-after images in ads for diet products are faked; the "before" image is often actually the "after," with the model having been instructed to gain fat for the "before" shot. Other times, as with certain celebrity-endorsed fitness products, the testimonials are paid for by the company selling the product, and the celebrity is endorsing the product because it's a "gig," not because of firsthand experience with its effectiveness.

Statistical Variation (Seeing the Forest from the Trees)

Another potential detour on the road to truth is the nature of statistical variation and people's tendency to misjudge through overgeneralization. Often in the fitness world, someone who appears to have above-average physical characteristics or capabilities is assumed to be a legitimate authority. The problem with granting authority to appearance is that a large part of an individual's expression of such above-average physical characteristics and capabilities could simply be the result of wild variations across a statistical landscape. For instance, if you look out over a canopy of trees, you will probably notice a lone tree or two rising up above the rest—and it's completely within human nature to notice things that stand out in such a way. In much the same manner, we take notice of individuals who possess superior physical capabilities, and when we do, there is a strong tendency to identify these people as sources of authority.

To make matters worse, many people who happen to possess such abnormal physical capabilities frequently misidentify *themselves* as sources of authority, taking credit for something that nature has, in essence, randomly

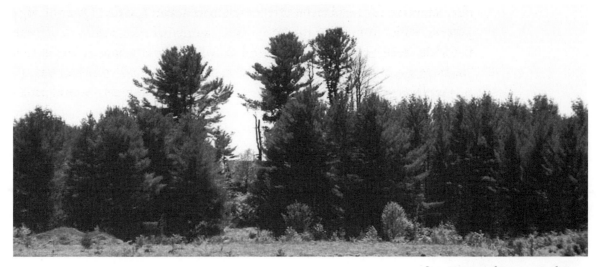

In a canopy of trees, random statistical variation allows some trees to stand out above the rest. A similar phenomenon allows certain members of the human species to display exceptional physical capabilities and distinctions. That most members of the species don't possess.

dropped in their laps. In other words, people are intellectually prepared to overlook the role of statistical variation in attributing authority.

This human tendency to misapply our cognitive generalizing capabilities in the face of statistical rarities has been explored in detail in books such as *Fooled by Randomness: The Hidden Role of Chance in the Markets and Life* (2nd Edition, Random House, 2005) and *The Black Swan: The Impact of the Highly Improbable* (Random House and Penguin Press, 2007), both by Nassim Nicholas Taleb. As used by Taleb, a "black swan" is a freak, random variation occurring in nature that people immediately seize upon—analogous to the tall tree sticking up out of the canopy. They then attempt to formulate a rational explanation to account for its existence. The usage derives from an old Western belief that all swans were white, because no one had ever seen a black one. When a black swan was discovered in seventeenth-century Australia, the term came to be associated with something that was perceived to be impossible but that actually came into existence.

This concept of statistical variation applies not just to physical attributes, such as athletic ability, muscle size, or height, but also to phenomena such as the marketplace. Taleb cites the wild success of the search engine Google as an example of a black swan in the business world. When people see such a tremendous business success, they are compelled to ask, "How did that happen?" The founder of the business naturally believes at some level that he or she did have a mechanism for achieving this amazing milestone. In some instances, the founders will endeavor to explain their method to anyone willing to pay to hear about it. The problem is that a large part of *all* success is based on a huge statistical variation that has nothing necessarily to do with a direct cause and effect.

That is why one can find "experts" offering contradictory advice on almost every subject, including health and fitness. In essence, what you have are two (or more) different trees sticking out of the canopy, and they have risen to such impressive heights not because of anything they did or did not do, but because of a statistical variation that gave them this advantage. In fact, what these two anomalies actually *did* may have been two entirely different things, but because they were both naturally predisposed to have success in this realm, they were likewise predisposed to make the same cognitive mistake of thinking, "What I *did* caused this to happen"— even if the techniques that these two people employed were diametrically opposed.

This state of affairs is not necessarily a deception on anyone's part; it's a natural mistake of the human cognitive process, because this process is set up to make generalizations and wide inferences based on observed data. Most of the time, this approach has proved to be an effective means of finding out what works—but it's most accurate when applied to the forest and not to the trees standing out above the canopy. The tricky thing to keep in mind, therefore, is that if you earnestly seek truth, you have to look for what is going to work for the *majority* of the population, rather than just the genetic exceptions. When scientific studies are conducted to try to establish such an explanation, the findings can be misleading if the study happens to include one or more of these genetic anomalies. That point brings us to the concept of standard deviation.

THE STANDARD DEVIATION

A standard deviation can be defined as the square root of the mean divided by the degree of variation off of that mean. So, one standard deviation from the mean to the left or to the right on the average bell-shaped curve will incorporate 85 percent of a given population. If you go two standard deviations off the mean, you are then incorporating 95 percent of that population. Out on the extreme ends at either side of the bell curve, you have figures of 2½ percent—that is, 2½ percent that are two standard deviations *above* the mean, and 2½ percent that are two standard deviations *below* it.

Most studies base their statistics on a Gaussian bell-shaped curve and Bayesian analysis. As a result, a problem arises when an anomaly is a factor. For example, including individuals such as a Mark McGwire, Sammy Sosa, or Barry Bonds in a study on training to improve performance in baseball, or including Bobby Orr, Wayne Gretzky, or Sidney Crosby in a similar study on hockey, would completely skew the results. In comparing their capabilities with those of the average baseball or hockey player, calculations will show that these individuals are roughly seventeen standard deviations away from the mean. If a researcher were to accidentally include just one of these bell-curve blowers in a set of statistics, the calculated mean would be thrown off three or four standard deviations to the right of where it should be. This is why in the world of fitness and muscle building, where one routinely reads articles detailing the training program of a given "champion," such recommendations have "zero" relevance to the average trainee.

To confound matters more, there is no shortage of people in the health and fitness industry who understand these facts and view them as a magnificent opportunity to deliberately defraud others and line their own pockets. Exploiting people by getting them to base their expectations of their training results to the right of the mean of the bell curve creates a scenario whereby marketers can say, "The element that *this* champion has that you don't is *this* product."

ASSUMING A CAUSAL RELATIONSHIP BETWEEN ACTIVITY AND APPEARANCE

You've probably heard the following type of advice: "Do you want to have the long, lean muscles of a swimmer? Then swim! Don't lift weights—you'll look like a bodybuilder!" Such claims are made all the time, and, despite their proliferation, they're wrong. Once again, you can chalk it up to the way the human mind operates. People will see a group of champion swimmers and observe a certain appearance, or they'll see a group of professional bodybuilders and observe another appearance, and it seems logical to assume that there is something about what these athletes are *doing* in their training that has created the way they appear. However, this assumption is a misapplication of observational statistics.

If you should ever attend a national AAU swim meet and sit through the whole day's competition, from the initial qualifiers to the finals, you would see these "swimmer's bodies" change dramatically over the course of the day. This speaks to the fact that it isn't the activity of swimming, per se, that produces this "type" of body; rather, a particular body type has emerged that is best suited for swimming. In other words, the genetic cream rises to the top through the selective pressure of competition. Competition, it can be said, is simply accelerated evolution.

The swim meet starts with the qualifying round. Perusing the people who are up on the blocks prior to the firing of the starter's pistol, you will note a broad array of body types. When the quarterfinals roll around, those body types will begin to resemble each other. When you get to the semifinals, they will look *very* similar, until finally, the competitors standing on the starting blocks during the championship look like clones. The reason? A self-selection process: accelerated evolution.

However, most of us simply watch the finals and see a group of people who look almost identical in terms of their body type competing in the same activity, and we conclude that this particular activity produced this body type. Thus, we draw an inference that is invalid because we are lacking a broader context, which in this instance should have included all of the different body types that also trained and engaged in the event. This is why you will hear people saying that you "ought to enroll in a Pilates class, so that you will develop a dancer's body," or you "ought to take dance aerobics classes, so that you will develop a dancer's body," or you "ought to take up swimming, because you want long, lean muscles, not big, bulky muscles." Such statements are the result of misapplied observations and of assumed cause-and-effect relationships that are actually inverted: it wasn't the activity that produced the body type; it was the body type that did well in that activity. It is the genetic endowment that produces the body type. Therefore, if one desires to have the body type of, say, a champion swimmer, the best course is to start by having the same parents as that champion swimmer—rather than his or her training methods.

THE DANGER OF ROMANTICIZING OUR ANCESTORS

In our species' evolutionary history, health and normal physiological functioning were always pinned to activities that maintained an appropriate balance between an anabolic (building up) state and a catabolic (breaking down) state. For most of our ancestors, that catabolic state was produced by a type of activity that was extremely high force, such as moving boulders, building fences, and hunting and gathering. What needs to be pointed out is that from the vantage point of DNA, the human body can be likened to a leased vehicle by which DNA is carried forward into the future. All DNA cares about is that you live long enough to procreate and raise children, who will, in turn, represent additional leased vehicles to carry on the DNA line. Once your DNA has been passed on to younger, fresher bodies, your body and its state of health and fitness are of little concern to your DNA. As for exercise, the *minimum* amount of physical activity that will stimulate the production of optimal health necessary for passing on DNA is what laid the foundation of your genome and how it responds to exercise.

While we tend to regard our ancestors as being far more active than ourselves and as being a group that ate "natural" foods and, consequently, enjoyed much better health than we do in the twenty-first century, the fact is that our ancestors' life expectancy up to the beginning of the twentieth century was the ripe old age of forty-seven.[1] Although a large portion of this shortened life span can be accounted for by illness, injury, and perinatal mortality, a lot of it can be attributed to the increased activity in which our ancestors had to engage in their search for food, which upset the delicate balance between the catabolic and anabolic states. It may be true that our evolutionary ancestors were far more active than their present-day counterparts, but it's also true that by the time most of them reached their early forties, their bodies were crippled by osteoarthritis and other wear-and-tear issues.[2]

As a result, it would be a mistake to look to the past in matters of health and fitness as a standard for modern expectations. Yes, our evolutionary past determined what an appropriate activity level is for our species today, but we also have to concede that, unlike our ancestors, we now have the knowledge necessary to bring the intensity of our physical activity up to a level that stimulates optimal health and enhanced fitness in such a manner that we won't have to suffer the same wear and tear that our ancestors did. We now know how to apply the right kind of physical activity that will bring forth a balance of the catabolic and anabolic states, a type of activity that will enhance our fitness without undermining our health.

Doctors and the Standard Deviation

It is a common practice to "seek a doctor's advice" regarding what type of exercise program one should follow to be healthy. This seems to most of us a logical thing to do. However, a legitimate problem can arise when soliciting the opinion of a physician on what fitness approach one should employ to optimize health, owing to the fact that physicians live and operate in a world of *pathology* that is so far to the left on the bell curve of health that many can't understand the concept of what is sitting at the mean. Because doctors (one of the authors included among them) deal on a daily basis with people who are *not* healthy, accurately assessing the links between exercise activity, fitness, and health can be difficult.

Because medicine by its very nature operates to the far left of the mean (over in the 2½ percent area), the average physician has no experience interacting with the other 97.5 percent and is therefore not in the best position to make assessments for the nondiseased population regarding how health and fitness are linked.

Be Cautious with Studies

So, if friends, relatives, doctors, champions, and popular publications are suspect, where can we turn for our answers? It's tempting to reply, "To science." However, even in this realm, one has to be careful to look closely at the studies that have been conducted, as not all studies represent an honest attempt to find the truth (and, as noted earlier, some are not performed properly). One should never, for example, skim through a study and just look at its abstract and conclusion sections (which, incidentally, is what most people do), because that's where one can get misled a lot of times.

The abstract and the conclusion can be supported by statistics that include curve blowers who skew the data. This occurs frequently in the medical literature, and drug companies take advantage of this situation by touting conclusions that are supported by skewed statistics. It's important to look at both the literature and how the data were collected. One may find that the actual data do not necessarily support the conclusion of a given study.

In citing studies in this book, we have endeavored to weed out the invalid from the valid, removing from consideration studies that contain the odd curve blower in favor of ones that are generally applicable to most potential readers. We did not undertake this enterprise with any preconceived notion of what we were going to find, but we at least knew what we were looking for in a valid study. The methods employed in looking for answers must be valid: the studies should be randomized and, where possible, double blind, so that there has been some sort of placebo control put into effect (this can be hard to do with physical training literature). These criteria are the hallmarks of valid studies. Disclosure of who funded the study is another consideration. If, for instance, a pharmaceutical company or a supplement company funded a study, any data derived may be suspect, and serious doubt will have been cast on its conclusions.

By actually looking at the data contained in these bona fide studies, we are better able to ascertain if the studies' conclusions are supported by their respective data and what their conclusions mean to the average person desiring valid information on health, fitness, and longevity.

Defining *Health, Fitness*, and *Exercise*

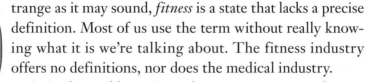

Strange as it may sound, *fitness* is a state that lacks a precise definition. Most of us use the term without really knowing what it is we're talking about. The fitness industry offers no definitions, nor does the medical industry.

A similar problem arises when one attempts to obtain a valid definition of *health*. In preparing to write this book, we looked extensively into the scientific literature, including many medical textbooks, to seek out a definition. We were surprised to discover that the terms *health* and *fitness*—while bandied about liberally within the fields of medicine, health care, and physical training—have never been given a universally agreed-upon definition. When examining his textbook from medical school, *The Pathologic Basis of Disease*, Doug discovered that while this book had no difficulty defining *pathology*, it never once presented a definition of *health*.

THE BALANCE OF CATABOLISM AND ANABOLISM

People routinely refer to *health and fitness* as if the two concepts were cojoined. The popular assumption is that as one's level of physical fitness rises, the level of health rises along with it. Unfortunately, no direct scientific link between these two conditions exists. The human body, you see, is never static; it is a dynamic organism that carries on a perpetual balancing act between breaking down (catabolism) and building up (anabolism). This is how your blood-clotting system functions, for example. It is continually breaking down and building up clots, keeping a balance between your blood viscosity and coagulability to ensure a smooth flow and still stem any bleeding that should occur (but not so aggressively as to produce clogged arteries and infarcts). Your pH balance, blood gases, hormone levels, electrolytes, fluid levels, and innumerable other complex processes are constantly shifting and changing as well within these catabolic and anabolic processes. Life, in essence, depends on this precise balance between a catabolic state and an anabolic state, and this balance is what defines the health of the organism.

In brief, these states can be summarized as follows:

Catabolic: Anything that results in the breakdown of the organism.
Anabolic: Anything that results in growth and differentiation of the organism.

Looking back at our species' hunter-gatherer days, we know that there were long periods when starvation was a real threat. During those times, a catabolic state would have predominated. Despite the obvious negative effects, research into calorie restriction and life extension has revealed that during such catabolic states the vast majority of DNA repair occurs. The lesson here is that a catabolic state is a necessary component of health, rather than something to be avoided. Knowing this, we must factor the catabolic and anabolic processes into any definition of health that we create. Health implies a disease-free state, and so the definition must acknowledge this component as well. Thus, given the lack of a working definition from the fitness and medical worlds, we cautiously offer the following:

Health: A physiological state in which there is an absence of disease or pathology and that maintains the necessary biologic balance between the catabolic and anabolic states.

The body's ability to sustain this balance between the catabolic and anabolic states manifests in an ability to make adaptive adjustments, thereby allowing for survival. Each and every day, your body must face numerous challenges, such as exposure to the various elements, muscular exertion, and the presence of pathogens. If it does not successfully adapt to these challenges, it is ill equipped to survive. Fitness, then, can be said to be the body's ability to withstand, recover from, and adapt to environmental threats in the form of stress-producing agents that act upon the organism. Or, stated another way:

Fitness: The bodily state of being physiologically capable of handling challenges that exist above a resting threshold of activity.

What is exercise?

To fully understand the relationship among exercise, fitness, and health, it is necessary to know precisely what exercise is, as opposed to mere physical activity. The important distinction is that exercise is purposefully directed activity that stimulates the body to produce a positive adaptation in one's level of fitness and health. Physical activity in general, while yielding the potential to produce certain adaptations in one's fitness and health, can unfortunately also undermine one's health. Therefore, we advance the following as our definition of exercise based on known facts:

Exercise: A specific activity that stimulates a positive physiological adaptation that serves to enhance fitness and health and does not undermine the latter in the process of enhancing the former.

Thousands of activities are popularly thought of as exercise, ranging from walking and running to calisthenics, weight training, and yoga. However, many of these activities do not qualify as exercise by our definition, either because they are inefficient at stimulating the mechanical and metabolic adaptations necessary to benefit the fitness (and, to a large extent, the health) of our bodies or because their continued performance results in an undermining of bodily health.

It is for this latter reason that we must exclude activities such as jogging and running from being considered as exercise. This determination may be upsetting to some, particularly those who run or jog, but the hard truth is that those who select running as their modality of exercise are taking a huge risk. Studies have documented that 60 percent of runners are injured in an average year, with one running injury occurring for every one hundred hours of performance.[1]

The damage caused by running will often manifest after a period of fifteen to twenty years of performing the activity, such as when runners who started in early adulthood reach the age of forty or fifty and find that they are no longer able to climb a flight of stairs without their knees aching; or they experience difficulty in lifting their arms above head level because of osteophytes (bone spurs) that have formed in the shoulder joint; or they can't turn or bend anymore because of chronic lower-back pain. These are progressive conditions, rather than immediate ones, and are consequences of inappropriate activities and activity levels that are chronically catabolic and are performed far too frequently to allow an anabolic state to manifest.

Even activities that are considered "mild" can become problematic in this respect. For instance, the thousands of rotations of the shoulder and elbow joint that take place over a career of playing recreational tennis can lead to osteoarthritis, even though the actual weight being moved in a tennis racket is modest. Any activity that is highly repetitive has wear-and-tear consequences that will sooner or later override the body's ability to recover and repair itself. If these types of activities are performed frequently (many times a week), they will typically manifest sooner.

HEALTH AND FITNESS—
WHAT'S THE CONNECTION?

When we looked at the scientific literature, we found not only a lack of definition for *fitness* and *health* but also, and even more surprising, a minimal (at best) correlation between *exercise* and *health*.

Many people have it in their minds that athletes are healthy *because* they are fit. However, if you look across the board at the professional level of sport, and if you analyze the statistics and health profiles of these athletes, you will find that, while they have supranormal levels of fitness, the means they employ to achieve this level of fitness may actually undermine their health. Most athletes who compete at a world-class level do not achieve that level of world-class performance in a way that enhances their health, and this is simply because it is *not possible* to do so. This is particularly the case if the sport in question is looking for a level of physical performance that is not necessarily part of the natural evolutionary background of our species.

A classical example is the tale of Euchidas, which comes down to us from the famed Greek historian Plutarch (c. A.D. 46–A.D. 120). After a Greek victory over the Persians at the battle of Platæa in 479 B.C., Euchidas ran to Delphi and back:

> . . . Euchidas of Plaæa, who promised that he would fetch fire as quickly as possible, proceeded to Delphi. There he purified his body, and having been besprinkled with holy water and crowned with laurel, took fire from the altar, set off running back to Platæa, and arrived thereabout sunset, having run a distance of a hundred and twenty-five miles in one day. He embraced his fellow citizens, handed the fire to them, fell down, and in a few moments died.[2]

And then there is the oft-told legend of Euchidas's contemporary, another distance runner named Pheidippides, which was originally reported by the Greek historian Herodotus (c. 484 B.C.–c. 425 B.C.),[3] and transmitted to future generations by Roman historians such as Lucian (c. A.D. 125–

after A.D. 180).[4] According to the legend, a Greek runner by the name of Pheidippides ran in excess of 145 miles (from Athens to Sparta) in roughly twenty-four hours, which was quite a display of ultraendurance athleticism. Pheidippides followed up on this feat by running an additional twenty-six miles from Marathon to Athens to announce the Greek victory. When he reached Athens he proclaimed (depending upon which ancient historian you read) either "Nike!" ("Victory!") or "Be happy! We have won!" Regardless, the ending to this tale is the same as that of Euchidas's: Pheidippides then fell to the ground—dead.

It's little wonder that an athlete's health would be gravely impaired by such an activity. According to the account of Herodotus, in that first run, from Athens to Sparta, Pheidippides completed the equivalent of back-to-back ultramarathons totaling more than two hundred kilometers.

Even more mind-boggling is the fact that, rather than being put off the notion of running such distances because of the health dangers, people instead raise monuments to the memory of Pheidippides by staging "marathons" and even the International Spartathlon race, which has its athletes running over purportedly the same 147.2-mile route from Athens to Sparta. To no surprise, some modern extremists in the realm of fitness have either met the same premature end as their Grecian counterpart (such as the author and running guru Jim Fixx) or suffered a host of ailments that are not compatible with long-term health and survival. The scientific literature is filled with data that strongly make the case that long-distance runners are much more likely to develop cardiovascular disease,[4] atrial fibrillation,[5] cancer,[6] liver and gallbladder disorders,[7] muscle damage,[8] kidney dysfunction (renal abnormalities),[9] acute microthrombosis in the vascular system,[10] brain damage,[11] spinal degeneration,[12] and germ-cell cancers[13] than are their less active counterparts.

Unaware of the anabolic/catabolic relationship, or that the pursuit of fitness can result in decidedly negative health consequences, most people still associate fitness (or exercise) with health. Instead of recognizing health as a delicate balance of opposite yet interrelated processes, they believe it to be something that is expressed across a broad continuum that never caps out. They assume there are increasing degrees of "better" health, as opposed to picturing health as the absence of disease. In reality, fitness and health are not extrinsically linked; as one goes up, the other does not necessarily go up with it.

With the correct modality of exercise, health and fitness can in fact track along together, at least to a point. However, simply performing physical activity can create a physiological situation whereby fitness levels rise, but health actually declines. This is the consequence of attempting to drive a level of specific metabolic adaptation for fitness that results in an imbalance between the anabolic and catabolic states.

We evolved as an organism that had to expend energy to acquire energy. This was the work-based way by which we acquired food and shelter to survive. It required a minimal level of activity, with intermittent high levels of muscular exertion and intensity. A balance was struck between the catabolic state that was a by-product of the exertion necessary to sustain ourselves and the anabolic state of being able to rest and recoup the energy required to obtain the nutrition needed to fuel the activities involved in our survival.

Fast-forwarding to our present-day situation, rather than a food paucity, there is a food abundance, and laborsaving technology relieves us from needing to expend as much energy to obtain that nourishment. As a result, there has been a compromise in our health that is the exact opposite of the problem that the endurance athlete faces; that is, there is now a huge portion of the population whose physical activity is of such low intensity that catabolism doesn't occur to any meaningful extent. There is no mechanism by which to drive a physiological adaptation for health or fitness.

It has been assumed that physical activity, per se, is responsible for health enhancement, but that assumption is flawed at the core. Such "health" benefits as might occur result only from one's current activity levels being so subnormal compared with our species' DNA blueprint that even a slight increase in activity produces *some* improvement. Raising one's muscular effort from a near sedentary state to a level slightly closer to what our species' DNA has encoded over tens of thousands of years (and which has changed significantly only in the past forty or fifty years) is by no means an optimal route to health.

People who believe that there is a constant and linear relationship between fitness and health are akin to a person who decides to measure water levels while standing at the beach. He takes the first measurement at low tide. When he sees the tide turn, he takes another measurement and notes that the tide rose five feet in twenty minutes. He checks it again and discovers that it has now risen fifteen feet in thirty minutes. He then concludes that in two weeks, the whole continent will be underwater.

This is the nature of the mistake we make when we observe increased activity levels supporting a slight upward tracking in the improvement of health. Health *will* improve—but only up until it rises to a *normal* physiological baseline. One thing that quickly becomes apparent from studying the scientific literature on overly active groups such as extreme-endurance athletes is that, in their quest to achieve higher and higher tiers of dominance in their field by extending their physical activity level to its limit, it is entirely possible (and probable) that the methods they typically employ in their training, combined with the rigors of long competitive seasons, will result in serious compromises in their health and shortened life spans.

The good news is that science now has a better understanding of how the human organism adapts and recovers. With that understanding comes the knowledge that it is possible to participate in a form of exercise that produces supranormal levels of fitness *without* compromising health and that, in many ways, serves to enhance health. This *scientific knowledge* has been gained through rational analysis, understanding, and application, based on the variables of volume (amount of exercise), intensity (effort and energy expended), and frequency (how often the activity is performed). When applied to an exercise program, these findings can result in the achievement of supranormal levels of function, in terms of fitness, while simultaneously maximizing health so that it reaches its natural peak.

THE QUEST FOR LONGEVITY

As we grow older, we naturally desire to grow older still. In this pursuit, we associate life with health, and health with fitness. So, it seems natural to inquire as to what exercises, what nutritional supplements, and even what drugs are available to aid us in our goal of living longer. It should be acknowledged that longevity, as with fitness, is not necessarily linked to health. It can be, but the important thing to remember is that health is ultimately linked to DNA—the self-replicating molecule that creates our bodies. The purpose of the body from the DNA's standpoint is merely to function as a vehicle to carry it forward into the future.

In our species' hunter-gatherer days, health was important to the degree that it allowed us to survive, as what brought us down most of the time were environmental factors such as disease, predators, childbirth, and trauma. Those are events that occur irrespective of one's level of fitness. Only through the application of human intellect and technology did longevity ever become an issue, or ever have an opportunity to track along with health.

As we began to live longer, new problems developed, because we now found ourselves in circumstances that did not track with our evolutionary biology. One set of problems arose as a result of higher population densities. By our living together in cities and being in close proximity to many people, the rapid spread of plague was made easier. The invention of the sewer greatly enhanced our species' longevity, as it dealt directly with waste management and the problem of disease. The invention of the subway and other modes of public transportation further improved that situation by allowing people to live in a more dispersed environment, thereby mitigating the dangers of contagion. Thus, the principal source of improvement in our species' life expectancy at the turn of the twentieth century was not medical advances; it was technological advances that shaped our environment so that it was more in tune with our evolutionary past.

It was, in short, not a "fountain of youth," or a drug, or an exercise, or a supplement that significantly enhanced our species' mortality rate. The secret formula boiled down to the distance we could put between ourselves and contagious disease; combined with laborsaving technology and other advances, it enabled our life expectancy to soar over the past century. To some extent, there have been advances in medicine, but advances in medicine in terms of life expectancy pale in comparison with advances in engineering. Those advances improved our life expectancy much more than medicine ever could. And, as we've seen, attempting to run a marathon or become "ultrafit" may not be the answer either.

LOOKING TO THE PAST

It is common for people to think back to a period in their lives, typically around the age of eighteen, when they were more active and were coincidentally also at their peak of fitness and health and to believe it was that "certain something" they *did* that created an enhanced level of fitness, health, and well-being. It's an association that they perceive as causation, which isn't the case at all. They forget that at that point in time, they were getting stronger every year (up until roughly the age of twenty-five) as a natural result of the body's growth process.

In the not-so-distant future, we may be in a position where the issue of functional ability will apply not merely to people who live into their seventies and eighties but to people living to be 120 or even 150 years! If so, then we are going to want to enjoy fitness and health for an even longer period than we do currently. This will not happen, and quality of life will suffer, unless we learn to incorporate a form of exercise that produces desirable adaptations without the wear-and-tear consequences that are observable from the more prevalent approaches. Ultimately, we need to make a concerted effort to learn how to distinguish between fitness and health and must shift our focus from how much exercise we can endure to how little we precisely require to cultivate the positive fitness properties from exercise, thereby enhancing our species' chances for improved health and longevity.

Global Metabolic Conditioning

T wo men are working out on a Friday afternoon. One is jogging along the side of a road. Cars whiz by as he plods along his route. He's sweating liberally and breathing rhythmically. On Thursday, he jogged for three miles; the day before, he jogged five; on Tuesday, it was three miles; and Monday saw him hitting the pavement for six miles. Today, after his usual ten-minute warm-up of various stretching movements, so as to not pull anything while jogging, he's hoping to get five miles in and finish the week at twenty-two miles. In addition, just as it was on Monday and Wednesday, today is his day to strength train, which he'll do for one hour right after he finishes his jog. He's thinking that he might slow his pace a little bit today, maybe take a little longer to get the five miles in, because the last time he jogged a little faster, that old shin splint flared up a bit, leaving him too fatigued to work out comfortably. He also has to cool down afterward, so that will be another ten minutes of walking and stretching.

He's a little bit stressed today about being able to get all of this in over the next three hours. He will still have to get showered, drive home in time to pick up his family, and then drive across town to his daughter's dance recital. But, hey, health comes first. He decides to call his wife; she can take their daughter to the recital, and he'll "do his best" to get there on time. He rationalizes away that gnawing feeling that he really should be there for his daughter by telling himself that he can do only what he can do. He'll get there when he gets there. His time spent away from his family engaged in his health and fitness pursuit this week has totaled twelve hours, not including driving time.

The other man is at a strength-training facility, where he is completing the last repetition of a set of leg presses. He performed two other exercises prior to this one, spending ninety seconds on a chest press machine and three minutes on an overhead pulldown machine, and he's hoping to get three minutes on this set of leg presses as well. To the surprise of both him and his trainer, it takes him four minutes to reach positive failure on today's leg press exercise. As he doesn't rest between exercises, his actual training time today is eight and a half minutes. His trainer reviews his chart with him after the workout, which shows that his strength is up 20 percent on both the pulldown and the chest press, his leg strength is up 30 percent, and his leg endurance is up by 45 percent. "Great workout," his trainer says as the man heads out the door and back to work, "see you in another seven days!" His time spent away from his family engaged in his health and fitness pursuit this week has totaled eight and a half minutes, not including driving time.

These opposing scenarios illustrate how the face of fitness is changing. More people are adopting the latter approach, simply because they desire total fitness, and all the benefits that come with it, without all the negatives that occur in the first model, the largest negative being an irreplaceable loss of time. But you couldn't possibly improve your cardiovascular system by working out for only eight and a half minutes a week, could you?

Sure, you could. In fact, you could improve it—markedly—and many other elements of metabolism as well, by working out for six minutes a week, and perhaps less.

THE McMASTER STUDIES

On June 6, 2005, CNN reported on the startling (to some) findings of a McMaster University research group, proclaiming that "six minutes of pure, hard exercise once a week could be just as effective as an hour of daily moderate activity."[1]

The study, published in the *Journal of Applied Physiology*, revealed that very intense exercise resulted in unique changes in skeletal muscle and endurance capacity. Changes such as these were believed to require hours of exercise each week. According to the "Methods" section of the study:

> Sixteen healthy individuals volunteered to take part in the experiment. Eight subjects (including two women) were assigned to a training group and performed exercise tests before and after a 2-wk sprint training intervention. Eight other men served as a control group and performed the exercise performance tests 2 wk apart with no training intervention. We also obtained needle biopsy samples from the training group to examine potential training-induced adaptations in resting skeletal muscle. We did not obtain biopsies from the control group for ethical reasons, because other studies have shown no change in resting muscle metabolite concentrations or the maximal activities of mitochondrial enzymes when control subjects are tested several weeks apart with no sprint training intervention. All subjects were recreationally active individuals from the McMaster University student population who participated in some form of exercise two to three times per week (e.g., jogging, cycling, aerobics), but none was engaged in any sort of structured training program. After routine medical screening, the subjects were informed of the procedures to be employed in the study and associated risks, and all provided written, informed consent. The experimental protocol was approved by the McMaster University and Hamilton Health Sciences Research Ethics Board.[2]

The program required the subjects to perform either four or seven thirty-second bursts of "all-out" stationary cycling, followed by four minutes of recovery time, for a total time of either two minutes or three and a half minutes of exercise. This was performed three times a week for two weeks, for a total of either six minutes or ten and a half minutes of exercise per week. At the conclusion of the study, when the subjects were retested, it was found that the endurance capacity in the "sprint" group increased by almost 100 percent (going from an average of twenty-six minutes to fifty-one minutes), whereas the control group (who weren't by any means inactive during this period, as they were jogging, cycling, or performing aerobics, as noted) showed no change. The muscles of the high-intensity-trained group also showed a significant increase in citrate synthase, an enzyme that is indicative of the tissue's power to use oxygen.

An editorial that accompanied the report of the study in the same issue of the journal offered this overview:

> Recreationally active college students performed only 2–4 min of exercise per session and just six sessions over 2 wk. The remarkable finding of this study was that this small total amount of very intense exercise training was sufficient to "double" the length of time that intense aerobic exercise could be maintained (i.e., from 26 to 51 min). Although peak oxygen uptake was not increased, aerobic adaptations did occur within active skeletal muscle as reflected by a 38% increase in activity of the mitochondrial enzyme citrate synthase.
>
> This study is significant because it contains a "documented" first, and more importantly it serves as a reminder to the scientific community and society. It appears that this is the first scientific documentation that very intense sprint training in untrained people can markedly increase aerobic endurance and that the total "dose" of exercise over the 2-wk period, performed in six sessions, amounted to only 15 min. This serves as a dramatic reminder of the potency of exercise intensity for stimulating adaptations in skeletal muscle that improve performance and have implications for improving health. In other words, we are reminded that intense sprint interval training is very time efficient with much "bang for the buck."

The findings of Burgomaster et al. challenge the concept that aerobic endurance performance is only enhanced by aerobic endurance training. On the surface, this concept seems logical, but it has been long ago proven wrong both in the realm of athletics as well as muscle biochemistry.[3]

Given that the study was conducted at McMaster University, in Canada, Martin Gibala, one of its lead researchers, was sought out by the national Canadian news network, CTV, for comment. "We thought the findings were startling," Gibala told CTV, "because it suggests the overall volume of exercise people need to do is lower than what's recommended."[4]

A SECOND STUDY

Still, a hue and cry arose from the fitness world, and even from some parts of the medical world. After all, these results were obtained in contrast with a control group that did not perform any specialized "cardio" training. Certainly, if a similar study were performed contrasting the benefits of the six-minute-per-week group with one that engaged in more traditional cardio modalities, the advantage would have to fall to the latter group. Gibala and associates in fact went back into the lab and performed another study that tested and examined changes in exercise capacity (muscular endurance) as well as molecular and cellular adaptations in skeletal muscle after subjects performed either high-intensity exercise (what they deemed a low-volume sprint-interval training, or SIT, group) or a more conventional endurance exercise (what they deemed a high-volume endurance training, or ET, group).

This time, their study again involved sixteen subjects, the average age of which was twenty to twenty-two years. All of the subjects were tested to see how long it took them to cycle 18.6 miles on a stationary bike. The subjects were then split into two groups and made to exercise at either high intensity with shorter volume or low intensity with higher volume, as determined by their maximum aerobic capacity (VO_2 max). The first group performed high-intensity work on a stationary bike—thirty seconds of intense bike riding (at 250 percent of their VO_2 max), followed by four minutes of rest. They repeated this procedure three to five times, until they had completed a total of two to three minutes of hard cycling. The second group took a more traditional approach, cycling at a moderate level (65 percent of VO_2

max) for 90 to 120 minutes. Both groups were made to cycle on three nonconsecutive days per week for a total of three "workouts" a week, or six total "workouts" performed over a two-week period. This made for a total of six to nine minutes of actual training time per week for the high-intensity group, versus four and a half to six hours for the higher-volume group, or twelve to eighteen minutes of total exercise for the high-intensity group and between nine and twelve hours of total exercise for the conventional (or low-intensity/high-volume) group over the same two-week period. After the two weeks of the program had elapsed, both groups were made to repeat the initial 18.6-mile cycling test.

Despite the fact that the more conventional endurance exercise group spent 97.5 percent more time engaged in exercise, both groups of subjects were found to have improved to the same degree. Note that the group that exercised 97.5 percent more did not receive an equivalent benefit from having done so. In fact, they received "zero" additional benefit from all of the extra time they spent engaged in exercise. Even in terms of endurance benefit, when the researchers performed muscle biopsies and further tests to determine changes in the subjects' fitness levels at the end of the two weeks, these tests showed that the rate at which the subjects' muscles were able to absorb oxygen also improved to the same level. According to the experimenters:

> Biopsy samples obtained before and after training revealed similar increases in muscle oxidative capacity, as reflected by the maximal activity of cytochrome c oxidase (COX) and COX subunits II and IV protein content (main effects, P 0.05), but COX II and IV mRNAs were unchanged. Training-induced increases in muscle buffering capacity and glycogen content were also similar between groups (main effects, P 0.05). . . .

This led the researchers to conclude:

> Given the large difference in training volume, these data demonstrate that SIT is a time-efficient strategy to induce rapid adaptations in skeletal muscle and exercise performance that are comparable to ET in young active men.[5]

In other words, there is *no* additional advantage in devoting hours per week to the pursuit of health and fitness improvement. Indeed, there is no additional physiological advantage afforded to one's body, including endurance or cardio benefits, by training that lasts more than six to nine minutes a week. Given the considerable wear-and-tear costs that attend exercise in general, particularly in activities such as running, the idea of increasing your risk of incurring such trauma is pointless from a health and fitness standpoint. The key findings in these studies indicate that in terms of overall health, a workout requiring six to nine minutes a week produced the same muscle enzymes (which are essential for the prevention of type 2 diabetes) as a workout requiring four and a half to six hours per week.

That is significant in light of the growing levels of unfitness. After the study, Professor Gibala stated, "We thought there would be benefits but we did not expect them to be this obvious. It shows how effective short intense exercise can be."[6]

MECHANICAL WORK IS MECHANICAL WORK

Your heart and lungs cannot tell whether you're working your muscles intensely for thirty seconds on a stationary bike or working them intensely on a leg press. The heart and lungs know only about energy requirements, which they dutifully attempt to meet. Four thirty-second intervals of high-intensity muscular exertion is four thirty-second intervals of high-intensity muscular exertion, whether that takes place exclusively in the lower body, as in stationary cycling, or in both the upper and lower body, as in resistance exercise. In either scenario, it is mechanical work by muscles that is the passkey to the aerobic and other metabolic machinery within the body's cells.

Shortly after these landmark studies were published, we contacted Martin Gibala to inquire at what trigger point in the workout sessions he believed the stimulus for these positive adaptations was imparted—after the first thirty-second interval, after the second, and so forth—and whether the same benefit might have been produced by working out with even less frequency, such as once every seven days. He responded that the minimum stimulus for adaptation might well have been even *less* than what was performed in his study.

Despite these facts, many skeptics will be left wondering how this could be. How could so little time spent exercising produce the same aerobic effects as more conventional workouts in only about 2 percent of the time? The answer is simple: high-intensity muscular effort.

THE CARDIOVASCULAR CONTINUUM

Cardiovascular exercise is frequently referred to as "cardio" or "aerobics." Dr. Kenneth Cooper, the physician who introduced the concept of "aerobics" to the world with his book of the same title, wrote a follow-up tome entitled *The New Aerobics*. In it, he recounted his experience with two individuals who came to him for a personal fitness assessment, which he conducted at his institute in Texas. Both clients had followed his prescription of performing a two-mile run five times a week, so he expected both individuals to be in similar condition. He was shocked to learn that one individual was in good shape and the other was not. "Why the difference?" he wondered. He recounted:

> I was perplexed until I asked another question: "How fast did you run your two miles?" The first said he averaged between 13:30–14:00 minutes whereas the second took over 20:00 minutes. One was a runner and the other a jogger. It was readily apparent that I needed to consider a factor other than distance—the time.[7]

Cooper then concluded, "You achieve a greater training effect if you put more effort into your exercise."[8]

As it turns out, Cooper had plunged in at the middle of a broad continuum and never pulled back far enough to take in the bigger picture and the full significance of what he was observing. He said that fourteen-minute two-mile runs produced better fitness results than did twenty-minute two-mile runs because the "training effort" of the muscles and the energy systems that serve them is harder in the former than in the latter.

However, it was the *harder* work of the muscles that resulted in the better improvement—and the shorter duration of the activity—not the activity itself. A twenty-minute two-mile run, for instance, would prove to be a better cardiovascular stimulus than would a two-mile run that took thirty minutes to complete. At the other end of the spectrum, an exercise that you're capable of performing for only sixty to ninety seconds will produce an even better cardiovascular stimulus, for the exact same reason: the muscles are working harder, as are the energy systems that support them.

To further illustrate, let's say you were able to perform a leg press exercise for fourteen minutes and then stopped—not because you had exhausted your leg muscles' fibers and energy reserves, but simply because an arbitrary number of minutes had passed (in this case, fourteen). You can well imagine how little stimulus in relation to your potential was actually provided, not only for your muscles but also for the energy systems, such as the aerobic system, that support the working of those muscles.

If the intensity of exercise is too low, nothing much in the way of a stimulus is presented to the body. On the other hand, if the intensity is too high in an activity such as running, you will increase the stimulus for positive adaptation, but you will also appreciably increase the chance of doing damage that will undermine your health. Here's the central message: what imparts the benefit—the stimulus to which the body adapts—is an aggressive recruitment and momentary weakening of muscle fibers. If you are able to recruit, fatigue, and weaken muscle fibers within a defined time frame, then you are going to recruit all of the different muscle fiber types aggressively and therefore get the most mechanical and metabolic effect for producing an adaptation. If the exercises are performed properly—that is, in accord with muscle and joint function—you can do so in a way that eliminates all of the other extraneous components, such as excessive force and excessive wear and tear on the joints, which are completely unnecessary for the delivery of the stimulus.

To understand why so many people believe that steady-state, low-intensity activity (and *only* steady-state, low-intensity activity) can produce aerobic adaptations and benefits to the human cardiovascular system, it's necessary to look back to how this belief originated. It is a fairly recent phenomenon, as is the entire field of coronary disease and problems.

THE QUEST TO UNDERSTAND THE HEART

William Harvey (April 1, 1578–June 3, 1657) was an English medical doctor who is credited with being the first to correctly describe, in exact detail, the properties of blood circulation throughout the body via the heart, arteries, and veins. Although a Spanish physician, Michael Servetus, discovered circulation a quarter century before Harvey was born, all but three copies of his manuscript, *Christianismi Restitutio*, were destroyed, and the secrets of circulation thus were lost until Harvey rediscovered them nearly a century later.

While Harvey discovered the exact means by which the heart circulates blood throughout the arteries and veins, the term *heart attack* was not described as a clinical entity until some three hundred years later, in 1912. Soon after, physicians everywhere became aware of its existence. When reflecting on his early years in practice, Paul Dudley White, an outstanding cardiologist of the mid-twentieth century, noted that before 1920, heart attacks and other symptoms of coronary atherosclerosis were relatively uncommon. In reviewing his earliest office records for telltale signs of heart disease, he did not see them occurring with any frequency.

From this little history lesson, it is clear that knowledge of the exact mechanisms of how the heart works, and how blood is circulated, is a relatively recent development in human history, and how to enhance its performance is an even more recent development. There were stops and starts in the speculation on how the cardiovascular system functioned. Servetus, who lived from 1511 to 1553, was believed to have based his conclusions on the works of Ibn al-Nafis, who lived from 1213 to 1288. Galen, a Greek physician and writer born in A.D. 129, was said to have advanced theories himself, more than a thousand years prior to this. Likewise, there have been similar stops and starts, as well as errors, in the advancement of knowledge of proper exercise to stimulate cardiovascular improvements in the human body.

The first attempt to confine an adaptive-specific exercise-response relationship to the aerobic system gained popular acceptance in the mid-1960s and was formulated by Kenneth Cooper. Again, though, while Cooper brought forth some important exposure for cardiovascular fitness and a means by which a successful measure of this fitness could be induced, he nevertheless plunged in at what we now know to be the middle of a rather broad continuum, and his prescription has created a situation by which individuals are seriously undermining other aspects of health in order to enhance one lone segment of it—the aerobic system. Rather than being known in the future as the man who "saved America's hearts," it is more likely that he will be regarded as the man who "destroyed America's knees."

Cooper started off the notion of "aerobics" as being synonymous with "cardiovascular" by attempting to produce a form of exercise that isolated the aerobic metabolic system. He believed that doing so would produce health benefits that were transferred to the cardiovascular system, and in a large measure, he was right. A lot of studies were conducted that appeared to confirm his premise, with the result that it soon became locked into the popular consciousness that "aerobic" equaled "aerobics," which equaled "cardiovascular conditioning." Over time, this belief has grown to such an extent that any activity—from walking, to jogging, to swimming, to cycling—that is low in intensity and steady in state is now referred to as "cardio."

The term *aerobics* is actually his creation. It is not really a word with any formal definition, but rather a noun used by Cooper to categorize his particular approach to training. *Aerobic*, in contrast, is a word that has a formal definition; it is an adjective that describes a particular metabolic pathway and means, literally, "with oxygen." The aerobic pathway is a segment of the totality of metabolism, but what is lost on many folks who exercise is that there are other metabolic segments as well that, collectively, work together to ensure the total health of the cell and, by extension, the health of the organism that the cells collectively work to support and sustain. Cooper believed (falsely, as it happens) that the aerobic subsection of metabolism was the most important—more important, in fact, than the totality of metabolic pathways that contribute to human functioning and health. He maintained that this one subsegment of metabolism could and should be isolated and trained. His belief in this regard has since been shown to be without foundation.

The first problem is the belief that the aerobic metabolic pathway can in fact be *isolated* from the rest of metabolism. The reality is that metabolism is an uninterrupted whole that is intrinsically tied together. The aerobic machinery is fueled by the substrate pyruvate, which can be produced only through the anaerobic pathway. Even at this most fundamental level, the interrelatedness of what Cooper believed to be antipodal elements of metabolism is self-evident.

How "cardio" really works

Figure 2.1 depicts a cell in the human body. The outer portion of the cell is filled with a fluid called cytosol. Inside this cell are little organelles called mitochondria. In looking at this image and at the nature of this process, you can see that there is no way that only *one* aspect of metabolism occurring in this cell is the exclusive domain of the cardiovascular system. In fact, the entire cell is connected to the cardiovascular system, and the extent to which you can ramp up all the components of metabolism is the extent to which the cardiovascular system will benefit. It does not benefit necessarily by any direct structural change within the cardiovascular system, per se, so much as it benefits through the metabolic adaptations that occur within the cell that the cardiovascular system supports. An examination of the following facts of metabolism will help to clarify this process.

Energy first enters into this cell in the form of glucose, a sugar derived from the breakdown of foodstuffs. (The body's preferred macronutrient for creating glucose is carbohydrate, but it can also produce its own glucose out of organic material if insufficient carbohydrate is ingested.) Once glucose has entered the cell, it is metabolized in the cytosol portion of the cell anaerobically through a series of some twenty chemical reactions until it becomes a chemical called pyruvate. This is an example of what is called "anaerobic" metabolism. Pyruvate then is moved inside the mitochondria, where it is metabolized through a complex process, making use of the Krebs cycle and respiratory chain. This process converts pyruvate to a total of thirty-six molecules of ATP (adenosine triphosphate, the currency of metabolism). This process is called "aerobic" metabolism.

While the Krebs cycle/respiratory chain can produce a lot of energy in the form of ATP, these pathways cycle slowly. By comparison, glycolysis—the process whereby glucose is metabolized in the cytosol to form

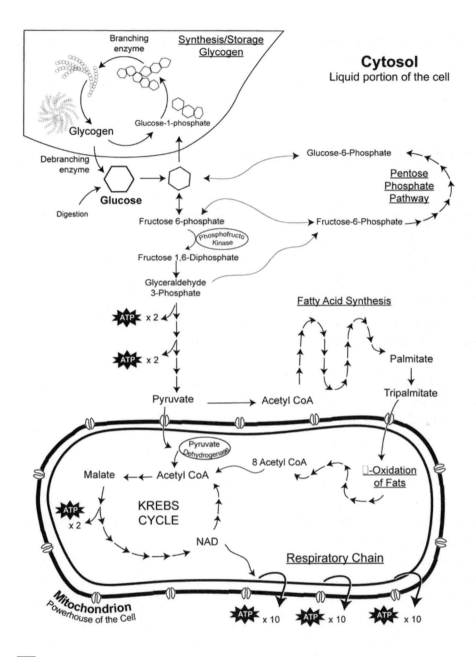

Cytosol
Liquid portion of the cell

FIGURE 2.1.

This overview of a cell in the body demonstrates the totality of metabolism that accompanies the performance of proper exercise and the integral role of the cardiovascular system.

pyruvate—produces only two molecules of ATP. However, the glycolytic cycle can turn at an infinitely faster rate than can the Krebs cycle/respiratory chain. Therefore, during life-or-death circumstances or extreme exertion, if you are well conditioned, you can turn the glycolytic cycle at an accelerated rate and supply energy needs for working muscles for a prolonged period. Because you are making pyruvate faster than it can be used by the aerobic cycle, the pyruvate begins to stack up and is converted by lactate dehydrogenase to a substance called lactic acid. (If this situation persists, you will produce lactic acidosis, or "lactic acid burn," in your muscles).

It is only by pushing the process of glycolysis to cycle as fast as it can (through anaerobic exercise) that you can produce pyruvate at a rate that causes the Krebs cycle to cycle as quickly as possible. If, for instance, you opt to perform low-intensity (submaximal) training, you will not be pushing your aerobic cycle as much as it can be pushed. Moving on, as you recover from high-intensity muscular activity, that lactate starts to stack up. The way the cell processes this lactate is to convert it back to pyruvate, which is the chemical form that allows it to be put into the mitochondria, where it is then metabolized *aerobically*. It is during "recovery" from high-intensity exercise that you're actually getting an increased stimulation of the aerobic system equal to or greater than what you would get from conventional steady-state "aerobic" exercise.

While many people have come to accept that the accumulation of lactic acid is a sign of an inferior aerobic pathway, the reality is that the glycolytic pathway will always be able to make pyruvate faster than the Krebs cycle can use it. The pyruvate dehydrogenase enzyme (which brings the pyruvate into the mitochondria for processing through the Krebs cycle) is what is called a "rate-limiting enzyme," which means that its rate of reaction is fixed. Therefore, it cannot be trained to improve its speed, which is always going to be slower than other metabolic steps in that cycle, irrespective of how "aerobically fit" you are. So, you're always going to produce lactic acid if you encounter meaningful muscular exertion. In other words, lactic acid is not an evil humor that you must avoid.

Moreover, if you have been subjected to proper physical training, you can actually make good use of the lactic acid that is produced. If you are intent on improving your aerobic capacity, it's important to understand that your aerobic system performs at its highest level when recovering from lactic acidosis. After your high-intensity workout, when your metabolism is attempting to reduce the level of pyruvate in the system, it does so through the aerobic subsegment of metabolism. It is also important to understand that since muscle is the basic mechanical system being served by the aerobic system, as muscle strength improves, the necessary support systems (which include the aerobic system) must follow suit. This explains why many middle-aged people and senior citizens note a profound lack of both strength and endurance when they suffer from a loss of muscle (a condition linked to aging and known as sarcopenia), as whenever a muscle's mass and strength are decreased, all of its metabolic systems downsize as well. This phenomenon carries profoundly negative health consequences.

THE CORI CYCLE

If our muscles require energy during high-intensity exercise or in an emergency, most of the ATP used will be derived from the rapid cycling of the glycolytic cycle. As this happens, lactate can quickly accumulate, but this is not necessarily the end of the road. Lactate formed during this process quickly diffuses from the muscles into the bloodstream, where it is then transported to the liver. In the liver, lactate is converted back to pyruvate, which is then reconverted to glucose by a process known as gluconeogenesis. The glucose thus formed is then transported out of the central vein of the liver and is made available for use again by the working muscles—or, if the exertion has ended, the glucose may then be stored as glycogen, which is simply a polymer, or "chain," of glucose molecules. This process is called the "Cori cycle." The enzymes and transporters of the Cori cycle are readily trainable by appropriate high-intensity exercise and have played a significant role in our species' survival, being a vital component of fight or flight. The survival and functional ability benefits of such conditioning are infinitely greater than those of pure aerobic conditioning, and yet almost nobody has ever heard of the Cori cycle.

THE BOHR EFFECT

As anyone who has ever visited a high-altitude site such as Denver will note, minimal exertion at high altitude will produce extreme shortness of breath. Within a few days of one's exposure to this environment, though, breathing will become easier. Most people assume in such instances that their breathing has improved because the oxygen pickup in their lungs has improved, but in actuality, they are breathing more easily because their oxygen pickup has *worsened*. The reason is that as oxygen diffuses from the lungs to the blood, it is picked up by hemoglobin molecules. Hemoglobin has a high binding affinity for oxygen and can therefore transport oxygen to the tissues where it is needed. The problem is that, on arrival at the tissue level, hemoglobin is reluctant to give up its oxygen. Your body, however, makes adaptations that decrease hemoglobin's affinity for oxygen in such a way that you can sacrifice oxygen uptake in the lungs (you generally have too much anyway) in order for you to have better delivery to the tissues. This is accomplished through a process known as the Bohr effect.

When you perform exercise of sufficient intensity to produce lactic acid, the resulting hydrogen ions are released in the blood and act on hemoglobin molecules to change their shape so that they have less affinity for oxygen. This results in improved oxygen delivery to the tissues. If you are exposed to repeated training at sufficient intensity, the effect is that you will synthesize a chemical called 2,3 diphosphoglycerate (2,3 DPG), which works like the Bohr effect but on a long-term basis. The 2,3 DPG is synthesized in elevated amounts in people living at high altitudes and in athletes who train repeatedly at levels of high intensity where the demand for oxygen delivery exceeds momentary capability for delivery. This is another metabolic adaptation that only high-intensity training can produce and that is infinitely important to survival and functional ability.

METABOLISM OF FATTY ACIDS

Excess energy is stored in the body in the adipocytes (fat cells) in the form of triacylglycerol. When energy is required under stress, such as during severe muscular exertion or during emergency situations, the hormones adrenaline and glucagon stimulate triacylglycerol mobilization by activating an enzyme called hormone-sensitive lipase. Figure 2.2 shows how hormone-sensitive lipase releases fatty acids into the blood, where they bind to a protein called albumin. Albumin transports these fatty acids to the muscles, where they undergo beta-oxidation to form thirty-five ATP molecules. Moreover, glycerol, an intermediate step in this process, can also be shunted to the liver and converted to glucose, which then can undergo further oxidation through a process that will yield an astounding ninety-six molecules of ATP. This is another aspect of metabolism that is developed only by high-intensity training, and it is also critical to both our survival and our functional ability. This should explode, forever, the myth that high-intensity training does not "burn fat."

GLYCOGENOLYSIS

High-intensity exercise also promotes glycogenolysis—the breakdown of glycogen for use as energy—within skeletal muscle. This is important for several reasons, the biggest of which is that it restores insulin sensitivity on muscle cells, which are the greatest glycogen depot in the body.

The average male human stores roughly 70 grams of glycogen in his liver and 210 to 220 grams in his skeletal muscles. (Females store about 20 percent less.) The glycogen that is stored in the muscles is for on-site use only, whereas the glycogen that is stored in the liver serves to maintain glucose homeostasis in the bloodstream (which is largely modulated on a long-term basis by a balance between insulin and glucagon). During our hunter-gatherer past, we (as is the case with most other animals) were at greatest risk of attack while feeding. Consequently, we evolved a mechanism by which we could turn our metabolism on a dime. The way this is accomplished is by the process of glycogenolysis within our skeletal muscles. In times of emergency, the glycogen that is stored within our muscles for on-site use is cleaved on the spot and quickly metabolized for energy within the cell from which it was cleaved.

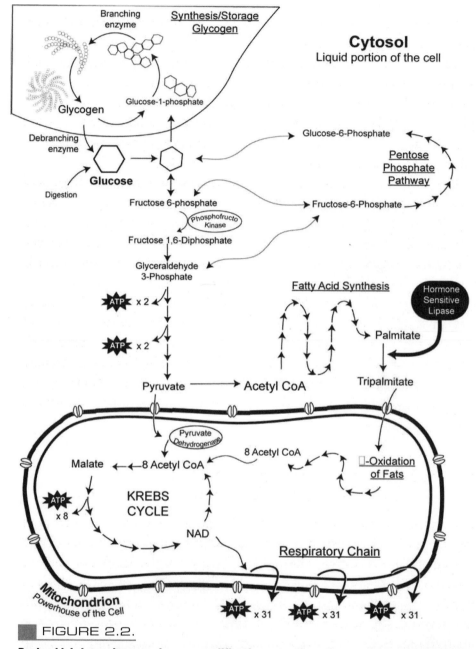

FIGURE 2.2.

During high-intensity exercise, an amplification cascade activates glycogen breakdown through debranching enzyme. The liberated glucose undergoes glycolysis and aerobic metabolism in the mitochondria to produce energy. Another amplification cascade acts on hormone-sensitive lipase, which releases fat for energy production in the mitochondria.

A similar process of tapping glycogen stores occurs during the performance of high-intensity exercise as a result of the fact that muscle fibers that would typically be called on only during emergencies (such as fight-or-flight situations) now have been activated, which, in turn, stimulates the secretion of stress hormones such as epinephrine and norepinephrine. When such an event occurs, the muscle cell empties itself of a significant amount of glycogen, which means insulin can now act on the cell surface, allowing glucose to reenter the muscle.

The same process that activates glycogenolysis also activates hormone-sensitive lipase and the mobilization of fatty acids for energy utilization. As a result, during high-intensity exercise, one is going to be mobilizing both glucose and fatty acids into one's bloodstream, where they then can be carried to the liver for beta-oxidation. They are then taken into the mitochondria to produce ninety-six molecules of ATP.

You often hear of people trying to restore insulin control "strictly through diet." This process is largely mediated through the balance of insulin to glucagon, and it will have to be followed on a long-term basis without the benefit of any amplification. The reason high-intensity exercise is so important for making such a dramatic metabolic shift is that it triggers both glycogen mobilization and hormone-sensitive lipase through what is called an amplification cascade.

THE AMPLIFICATION CASCADE

In an amplification cascade, rather than one molecule acting to produce one metabolic effect (such as one molecule of glucagon cutting in and causing the release of one molecule of glucose off glycogen), one enzyme instead activates another set of enzymes. It may activate ten or one hundred of the next step in the cascade. Each one of those one hundred enzymes in turn activates the next step of the cascade, and then each one of those one hundred that have been activated now activates another hundred, and so on down the line. So, instead of having to shuttle a glucose molecule off a glycogen chain one molecule at a time, you can have activity of an enzyme that is amplified exponentially, so that you're now cleaving thousands of molecules of glucose off simultaneously for emergency usage. The magnitude of glycogen emptying that occurs from muscle is greatly accelerated and expanded by this process.

An excellent explanation of this phenomenon can be found in the text-book *Metabolism at a Glance*,[9] which presents an amazing recap of how this huge energy release is set in motion by one molecule of adrenaline that serves to cleave thousands of molecules of glucose off of glycogen. An amplification cascade is thus extremely effective in supplying huge amounts of energy to our working muscles during an emergency situation by employing a series of enzymes that serve to amplify each other. Further, while this amplification cascade is breaking down glycogen for use, an enzyme involved with the formation of glycogen prohibits the body from synthesizing glycogen, so that now the body is employing all of its energy systems in the direction of glycogen breakdown and glucose utilization, with nothing moving in the direction of glycogen storage.

Sustained health benefits

It is by the process of glycogenolysis and the resulting amplification cascade that high-intensity exercise really taps into the largest store of glucose in your muscles and mobilizes it so that in the postexercise period, the result-ing glucose void must be filled or replenished. As a consequence, a situation has been created whereby the insulin receptors on the surface of the muscle cell now become more sensitive to aid in the process of replenishing this deficit. This replenishment period can last as long as several days, depend-ing on the depth of drainage. Insulin sensitivity is prolonged by the higher level of drainage that attends high-intensity training, as opposed to just an immediate, postworkout sensitivity boost. This replenishment process occurs by a standard glycogen synthesis pathway that does not involve a similar mechanism of amplification.

As insulin sensitivity is prolonged, enduring for several days afterward, the sensitivity is also heightened by the magnitude of the glucose that has been mobilized out of the muscle. As it's not a little amount of glucose that has been utilized (as would be the case with, say, a treadmill trek for thirty minutes at low intensity), but rather a lot that has to be put back into the muscle, the magnitude of this effect is exaggerated. What becomes important is not just the insulin-sensitivity issues but also the downstream metabolic effects of this process. For instance, if your glycogen stores are completely full, then you are in a situation in which glycolysis is inhibited by the stacking up of glucose within the body. (See Figure 2.3.) High levels of glucose produce high levels of metabolic by-products that then inhibit further use of glucose for fuel, which will trigger a situation in which you are now going backward up that metabolic pathway to synthesize more glycogen.

At the point that your glycogen stores become completely full, glucose cannot be rammed down the path of glycogen synthesis anymore. Therefore, its only metabolic destiny is now to be metabolized as fat. (See Figure 2.4.)

When glucose levels are high and your glycogen stores are completely full, the phosphofructokinase enzyme (which is involved in the metabolism of glucose) gets inhibited. The glucose can now go only to the level of fructose-6-phosphate on the glycolysis cycle, at which point it gets shunted over to the pentose phosphate pathway, which will then convert the glucose, through a series of steps, to glyceraldehyde-3-phosphate (also known as triose phosphate or 3-phosphoglyceraldehyde and abbreviated G3P), which is a fat precursor. Several more metabolic steps are then taken, the end result of which is the production of an energy-bearing chemical called NADH, which is used to fuel fatty acid synthesis. Full glycogen stores, if coupled with elevated carbohydrate levels, actually stimulate the production of fatty acids, particularly in the liver, which drives up the amount of very low-density lipoprotein, because that is the first thing that is converted from glucose to fats. That very low-density lipoprotein will be converted to LDL cholesterol, which is a marker for cardiac risk factors.

What this tells us is that low-intensity, steady-state (popularly referred to as "cardio") activity does not tap the fast-twitch muscle fibers that possess the most glycogen. Consequently, the muscles are never emptied of meaningful levels of glucose, with the result that the circulating glucose has nowhere to be stored—except as bodyfat. Moreover, the muscle cell walls lose their sensitivity to insulin but become inflamed by the high levels of insulin that the body has produced to deal with the high levels of circulating glucose. The body mortars this inflammation with LDL cholesterol, which puts the low-intensity exerciser at greater risk for cardiovascular

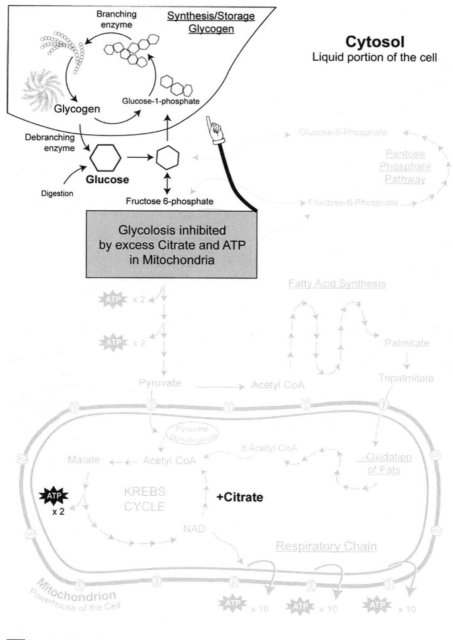

High glucose levels signal a high-energy state, which inhibits glycolysis and activates glycogen synthesis.

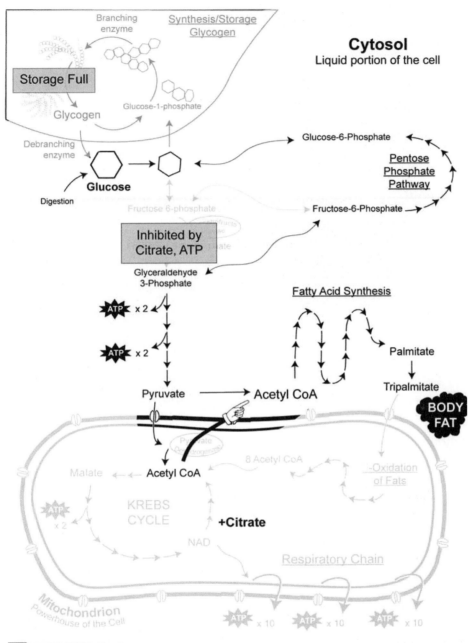

Cytosol
Liquid portion of the cell

FIGURE 2.4.

When glycogen stores are full, additional glucose gets shunted toward fat synthesis.

problems. It does sound contradictory, but the cell that is completely full of glucose/glycogen decreases its sensitivity to insulin to protect itself from more glucose being transported in, as excess glucose results in "glycosylation" of its machinery. It literally becomes a sticky mess. Metabolizing excess glucose produces oxidative free radicals that are highly inflammatory. Also, insulin is a hormone that stimulates inflammation, including inflammation on the arterial walls, which is patched by LDL cholesterol.

PREVENTING MUSCLE BREAKDOWN

High-intensity exercise is necessary to bring about the foregoing positive metabolic adaptations. Fortunately, the intensity level of high-effort muscular work requires only a brief duration of such exercise. If exercise is carried out for too long, glycogen begins to deplete, and protein from muscle tissue is used to maintain glucose homeostasis. Muscle tissue is broken down into its constituent amino acids and converted to glucose via the process of gluconeogenesis in the liver. Thus, if exercise is performed too long, as in ultraendurance events, extreme wasting of muscle tissue can occur.

It's even possible to perform a type of activity that is of insufficient intensity to bring about the desired metabolic adaptations yet is of sufficient volume to bring about large amounts of tissue destruction. This type of activity is called steady-state, or conventional, "aerobic" exercise. It cannot produce much in the way of metabolic adaptations, and its price is the destruction of the most productive and protective tissue of your body.

PERIPHERAL ADAPTATIONS

Let us suppose that you and an eighty-year-old man, who appears frail and atrophied, decide to walk up two flights of stairs. When you get to the top landing, you feel fine, while the elderly man is obviously winded. The reason for this difference in response is not that his heart and blood vessels are in worse condition than yours. It's really a matter of strength.

Given that individual muscle fibers make up motor units (as discussed in detail in Chapter 3), assume you have 2 units of strength per motor unit, while the elderly man's muscles have atrophied and withered over the years to the point where they have been diminished to 1 unit of strength per motor unit. For this example, let's assign the amount of work it takes to climb those two flights of stairs a numeric value of 200 units, meaning that it takes 200 units of mechanical work from the body's muscles for anyone to make it to the top of the stairs. Since your motor units have 2 units of strength each, your body will have to recruit only 100 motor units to accomplish this task, whereas the elderly man's motor units have only 1 unit of strength, so he has to recruit 200 motor units to accomplish the same task. Consequently, your cardiovascular system has to support the work of recruiting only 100 motor units, while his cardiovascular system has to support the recruitment of 200 units.

As you can see, the real cardiovascular benefit that can come from exercise is strengthening, so that, per unit of work that you do, the cardiac and vascular system will have to support a recruitment of a smaller number of motor units to accomplish a specific task. The real cardiovascular benefits from exercise, then, occur as a result of peripheral adaptations, not central adaptations.

How did aerobics catch on?

We now know that "aerobics" is a low-intensity form of physical activity that allows the mitochondria to do their work at a submaximal pace, with the upshot that only one aspect of metabolism—the aerobic system—is emphasized. Over several decades, all sorts of positive health benefits became associated with this specific metabolic adaptation. Soon, it became a foregone conclusion that aerobic conditioning *was* cardiovascular conditioning and that the two were interchangeable. What never seemed to have been pointed out is that the heart and blood vessels support the *entire* functioning of the cell, not just the mitochondria. *Every* component of metabolism is supported by the cardiovascular system.

Strength training is actually the best way to train the cardiovascular system precisely because, unlike what we refer to as "aerobics," strength training actually involves and stimulates all of the components of metabolism. This includes the metabolism that goes on in the cytosol (the liquid portion of the cell and in the absence of oxygen) *and* the metabolism that occurs in the mitochondria (i.e., in the presence of oxygen).

LOW INTENSITY (HIGH RISK) VERSUS HIGH INTENSITY (LOW RISK)

Let's return to the two hypothetical individuals working out in the example that started this chapter. One is going to perform steady-state, low-intensity running five days a week, and the other is going to perform high-intensity strength training once a week. The individual who performs the high-intensity training will be the one who gets the benefit of glycogen depletion and reloading, while the one performing the lower-intensity, more frequent steady-state work is at far greater risk for cardiovascular disease, particularly conditions resulting from increased cholesterol levels.

Not only is he *never* emptying his muscles completely of glycogen with his low-intensity, steady-state activities (in the pursuit, he believes, of improving his cardiovascular health), but also, because he is not using his muscles at a high enough level of effort, they will—as studies have shown—begin to atrophy. The glycogen-storing capacity of these muscles will diminish with each successive week that he engages in his low-intensity, steady-state activity, lowering the level at which a cell becomes "full" of glucose, and the bloodstream begins shunting the superfluous glucose to fat storage, thus hastening a process that could lead to coronary artery disease. His glycogen-storing capacity is also reduced, so that the point at which his muscles become completely full of glycogen—and, therefore, the point at which he will develop insulin resistance—will now potentially come sooner. This is particularly true if he experiences a loss of muscle mass, which low-intensity, steady-state activity can perpetuate.

The other factor to consider is that while the runner may be obtaining some benefit from his modality of physical activity as compared with someone who is completely sedentary, he is also plodding along in a kind of fool's paradise, because he's not even getting all of the aerobic benefits that he could be getting from exercise. In the process of doing what he thinks is correct, over the long term, he could actually be decreasing his muscle mass to the extent that his glycogen storage capabilities decrease, so that his risk for developing insulin insensitivity is going to rise.

Also recall that he is doing a type of activity that relies predominantly on the aerobic metabolic system, the primary form of metabolism of which is oxidative, meaning that it is going to produce more inflammatory free radicals than are produced by doing something that is briefer and of higher intensity. Moreover, because running for long periods burns primarily fat, technically, he's not tapping his glycogen stores to any significant degree, with the result that his insulin sensitivity is going to go down over time with this type of behavior. That's going to put him at increased risk for coronary disease—the very thing that he foolishly believes he is taking steps to alleviate by engaging in his low-intensity, steady-state activities.

HORMONE-SENSITIVE LIPASE

There is an assumption that low-intensity exercise is necessary for fat burning and also that it burns more fat than high-intensity exercise. The reality is that no exercise, per se, burns a lot of bodyfat. The average person weighing 150 pounds burns roughly 100 calories per mile—whether the person walks or runs that mile. Since there are 3,500 calories in a pound of bodyfat, it would be necessary to run or jog for thirty-five miles to burn 1 pound of bodyfat. While both low- and high-intensity physical activity burn calories, high-intensity exercise does something that is highly important in the fat-burning process that its lower-intensity counterpart does not: it activates hormone-sensitive lipase.

When we're mobilizing glycogen out of a cell during high-intensity exercise, we're also able to activate hormone-sensitive lipase, which permits the mobilization of bodyfat. If insulin levels are high, even in the face of a calorie deficit, hormone-sensitive lipase will be inhibited, and mobilizing fat out of the adipocytes will become essentially impossible. This may explain why people who diet and take up either walking or jogging often find it difficult to lose much in the way of bodyfat.

There are ways of getting around this predicament, however, one of which is by controlling insulin levels adequately such that serum insulin levels remain low. In this way, hormone-sensitive lipase is easier to activate, making mobilized bodyfat the body's primary energy source preferentially over other sources. This state can be achieved through a diet that is relatively restricted in carbohydrates, but one will have more dietary latitude if, in concert with going easy on the carbohydrates, one engages in the performance of high-intensity exercise. That's because in the face of high-intensity exercise (with its stimulation of adrenaline), hormone-sensitive lipase is operating under an amplification cascade similar to that which occurs with glycogen mobilization. Again, an excellent overview of this process is presented in the biology textbook *Metabolism at a Glance*.[10]

During the same time that glycogen synthesis is being inhibited, so, too, is fat synthesis being inhibited while fat is being cleaved. So, you're operating both on unplugging the drain and on turning off the faucet, so to speak; you're inhibiting fat synthesis while you mobilize fat, in the same way that you inhibited any glycogen synthesis while you were mobilizing glycogen. Both of these conditions occur under the event of high-intensity exercise, mediated via adrenaline through an amplification cascade, which magnifies the effect.

REEXAMINING "CARDIO"

Your cardiovascular system, it should be remembered, is always engaged. It's engaged when you are standing in a room talking to someone: your heart is beating, your blood is circulating, and your lungs are taking in air and expelling carbon dioxide 24-7. The only way to get your cardiovascular system to work harder is by performing mechanical work with muscle. Any increase in muscular demand simultaneously increases the involvement of your cardiovascular system to a much greater extent. So, you are always "doing cardio" in the popular sense of the term whenever you do anything—or nothing.

Given the interrelatedness of the various metabolic cycles, the notion that you can separate any of these metabolic cycles out from each other is erroneous; they are always running concurrently and together, though some of them can outpace the others. Anything that defines exercise from a metabolic sense is raising the intensity level above its baseline, and even if such pathways could be isolated, they shouldn't be if your goal is total health and fitness.

VO$_2$ MAX AND SPECIFICITY

It is true that in certain VO$_2$ max studies, cardiovascular improvement has been demonstrated to attend steady-state, low-intensity activity. The problem with VO$_2$ max testing is that when your only tool is a hammer, the whole world becomes a nail. A VO$_2$ max test is based on the assumption that the premise of aerobic exercise is correct—that somehow a specific type of metabolic work is linked to cardiovascular function. By the same token, if we were to assume that a different type of metabolic work is linked to cardiac function and then test for that, we could prove that assumption as well. If, for instance, we decided that it is your ability to metabolize lactic acid that is a marker of cardiac health, we could perform a test that involved measuring lactate utilization at high intensity and then run on the assumption that this links to cardiac health and thus reveal how high-intensity strength training is a superior means of producing lactic acid, metabolizing it, and, therefore, improving cardiovascular health.

Because the cardiovascular system is always going to be linked to any specific metabolic adaptation you make, your results are going to be tied to whether you want to make metabolic adaptations to low-intensity activity or high-intensity activity.[11] As we've seen, a whole spectrum of specific metabolic adaptations can be made with high-intensity training, so why would you limit yourself to only one aspect of metabolic enhancement?

As another example, if you simply wanted to improve someone's VO$_2$ max for walking or jogging on a treadmill, you could train this person in a steady-state fashion on a treadmill and test the subject's VO$_2$ max using a treadmill. As a result, you will show a marked improvement. Still, if you now test this person on a bicycle ergometer instead of the treadmill, you will find little or no improvement in VO$_2$ max.

An elegant study was performed in 1976 in which the experimenters recruited thirteen subjects and trained them on a stationary bike. However, they had them train only one leg; the other leg wasn't trained at all. The trained leg employed a sprint and/or an endurance (steady-state) protocol. The subjects performed four or five such workouts per week for four weeks. After the study, when the researchers tested the subjects' VO_2 max by having them repeat the exercise with the trained limb, they noted an increase in VO_2 max of 23 percent. This low-intensity, steady-state exercise was supposed to produce a central cardiovascular adaptation, but when the experimenters tested the subjects' untrained legs, they discovered that the untrained limbs showed no improvement in VO_2 max at all.[12]

This study established that what is being measured with a VO_2 max test is not a central cardiovascular improvement, but rather simply a specific metabolic adaptation that occurred at the muscular level. This also speaks to the fact that if you choose running as your exercise, any improvement in your VO_2 max will be restricted to your legs for the activity of running. It's not having a central adaptation, as the muscles in your trunk and arms will be largely unaffected, and the effect will not be transferable to any other exercise modality.

The Limited Specificity of Aerobic Exercise

I lived in Ohio for three years and, at the time, performed conventional aerobic exercise in conjunction with my strength training. Along with most other people in those days, I accepted it as something that I *had* to do. During the spring and summer, I would run outdoors on the road, but in the winter, I would run indoors on a treadmill at the gym where I worked out—in order to "maintain my aerobic fitness."

When springtime came around, I would do my first run out on the road, and I felt as if I was going to die while I was doing it. That's because the specific motor skill of running on a treadmill is completely different from running on ground. When you're running on ground, there's a two- or three-part component: foot strike, push-off, and then a recovery stroke, whereas on a treadmill, because the ground is spinning underneath you, so to speak, there is a foot strike, no push-off, and then recovery—so one entire component of the stride is missing on a treadmill run. The mechanics and the skill factor for running on the earth versus running on a treadmill are completely different.

Consequently, any metabolic adaptations that you thought you had suddenly seemed to disappear, even though the assumption was that you're producing some sort of central cardiovascular adaptation that ought to be transferable to any activity. Why it took me so long to make the connection that I was just making a specific skill-set adaptation with one activity that completely goes away when I performed another, I can't figure out.

Another pertinent example of the limited specificity of aerobic exercise occurred when I was in the air force in Ohio. The air force had these minimal fitness requirements that you had to meet every year, and the powers that be devised this silly formula for using an ergometer exercise bicycle to back-calculate your VO_2 max based on your heart rate at a certain workload.

Well, in my group, there were a couple of people who were competitive 10k and marathon runners who thought, "Oh, my aerobic fitness is great. I'll just show up and do the test." We also had an overweight and deconditioned fellow take part in the test who was very smart. In the two weeks leading up to when we had to have this test done, he went over to the gym every day after work and used the *exact* bicycle that was going to be used in the testing; he practiced his cycling against *exactly* the resistance that was going to be used for the testing, for the *exact* amount of time that the test would take. He got the highest score of anyone, and the two competitive runners who were supposedly extraordinarily aerobically fit failed the test.

The reason for this outcome was that the overweight fellow realized that what you had to do was train for the test in exactly the same way that you would be tested. You don't, for instance, go into a math test having studied only English beforehand, and he made that connection. As a result, an obese and deconditioned fellow, just by practicing the test, passed it with flying colors, whereas the people who believed that they already had this central cardiovascular adaptation and would ace it actually failed it. All they had gained through their efforts was a specific motor skill set or metabolic adaptation for running that did not transfer onto the bicycle.

—Doug McGuff, M.D.

In conclusion, we would ask you to consider the following three points:

1. Low-intensity, steady-state activity is not necessarily the best way to improve your cardiovascular system.
2. Other elements of metabolism apart from the aerobic system should not be ignored, but are when you employ a low-intensity, steady-state approach to exercise.
3. Legitimate health benefits are attainable from high-intensity exercise as it pertains to metabolism that are not possible from lower-intensity exercise.

Any positive adaptations made by the body as a result of the stimulus of exercise are metabolic improvements that occur in the muscle tissue itself. From a metabolic standpoint, what's going on in a muscle is partitioned from the rest of the body. That explains how an animal can have a form of metabolism running through the liver that's predicated on insulin and glucagon while it is eating and, in an instant, convert from an energy-storage mode to a metabolic process that is partitioned within the muscle and that results in massive energy expenditure. Such 180-degree turns in metabolic activity can take place only within muscle tissue, because that is where these processes exist.

The center of metabolic health, then, is not the heart and cardiovascular system; it is the muscular system. That's where the enzymatic activity takes place, and it takes place by means of an amplification cascade, so that when you activate the cause, the effect is much greater at the muscular level. It's in muscle where all the "gold" that can be panned from exercise is found. The fitness world's misplaced focus on the cardiovascular system needs to be redirected to the muscular system, because that's where everything that results in positive adaptive change happens.

The Dose-Response Relationship of Exercise

n the mid-1990s, author Doug McGuff was revisiting his pharmacological notes from medical school and discovered an interesting parallel between medicine and exercise. Both a drug and an exercise act as a stimulus to the body, both require an optimal concentration, both require a dose that is not "too high," and both require an appropriate dosing frequency.

The concentration of the drug is analogous to the intensity of the exercise, the dosage is analogous to the amount of sets performed in a given workout, and the dosing frequency is analogous to the frequency of exposure to the training stimulus. Also, just as with medicine, there exists in exercise a "narrow therapeutic window" within which the volume of exercise can act to stimulate the body to produce a positive adaptive response that is optimal. Transgress the borders of this window and, as with a drug, the benefits do not increase, but rather the toxicity does. The following sections outline each of these factors in more detail.

THE CONCENTRATION (INTENSITY)

In medicine, the potency of the drug is measured by its concentration. In exercise, the concentration or potency of the stimulus is determined by how many muscle fibers are called into play during the course of the exercise, with few fibers corresponding to a low concentration and many fibers corresponding to a large concentration.

It is the brain that recruits muscle fibers, but it does so solely as it perceives the need for them. This is accomplished via the central nervous system through motor nerves, which, in keeping with the dictates of the brain, follow a relatively fixed order in the recruitment process. The process involves only the precise amount of electrical current necessary to activate the amount of muscle fibers required to generate a specific amount of force.

Studies of human anatomy and physiology have isolated four distinct types of muscle fiber within our species. The breakdown is somewhat complicated, because within one main class (the fast-twitch), there are three subclassifications. To confound matters more, the classification schemes for muscle fibers have differed over the years, resulting in no fewer than three separate classifications for the same grouping. The classification of the four fiber types under these three schemes is as follows:

Classification of the Four Fiber Types

I	SO (Slow, Oxidative)	S (Slow)
IIA	FO (Fast, Oxidative)	FR (Fast, Fatigue Resistant)
IIAB	FOG (Fast, Oxidative, Glycolytic)	FI (Fast, Intermediate Fatigability)
IIB	FG (Fast, Glycolytic)	FF (Fast, Fatigable)

Fast-twitch muscle fibers differ from their slower counterparts in many ways, most notably in their endurance capacity. That is, it's in the endurance realm, rather than in the velocity or speed department, that their differences become most apparent. The fast-oxidative (FO, Type IIA) fibers have a poor endurance profile. (The modifier *oxidative* refers solely to the aerobic machinery within the fast-oxidative fiber itself.) The fast-glycolytic (FG, Type IIB) fibers have more power but are also poor in terms of their endurance capabilities. (The modifier *glycolytic* refers to the anaerobic machinery within the fast-glycolytic fiber itself.) Intermediate in speed, endurance, and power are the fast-oxidative-glycolytic (FOG, Type IIAB) fibers, which contain both the anaerobic and aerobic machinery within their cellular makeup. On the other side of the coin, slow-twitch muscle fibers (SO, Type I) are endurance fibers used primarily by people who engage in distance activities. They are powerful aerobically, with lots of aerobic enzymes, blood vessels, and myoglobin, which is an oxygen-storing endurance compound. The slow-twitch fibers, however, aren't capable of creating much force and, consequently, don't possess the inherent mass potential of their quicker-twitching cousins.

An individual's fiber type and distribution are genetically predetermined. Most of us are brought into the world with a relatively even distribution of all types of fibers. Of the four fiber types, the slow fibers are the easiest to engage, owing to the fact that they don't require a lot of energy, so the body doesn't hesitate in sending them into action. Slightly more energy is required to engage the FO fibers, and more still for the FOGs. The ones that require the highest energy to engage are the FGs. In line with our species' proclivity to conserve energy whenever possible, the brain will first attempt to contract against a resistance by recruiting only the slow fibers, which will prove inadequate for the task. The brain will then recruit the FOs and, shortly thereafter, the FOG fibers to assist with the task of contraction. If the weight is light or moderate, these are all the fibers that will need to be recruited. However, if the weight is heavy enough, a signal will be sent out to engage the elusive FG fibers.

This process is known in physiology circles as "orderly recruitment," in recognition that the brain does not engage in the firing of muscle fibers randomly. When recruiting muscle fibers for the purpose of contraction, the brain doesn't concern itself with speed; what it cares about is force. It has no interest in how fast you want to lift a weight or how quickly you wish to run. Again, it cannot randomly recruit muscle fibers. Instead, the brain ascertains the precise amount of force your muscles require to move a precise resistance and, accordingly, recruits the precise amount of muscle fibers necessary to do the job as economically as possible in terms of the body's energy systems.[1] (This occurs up to a certain threshold point; once this point is reached, increased force is produced by an increase in the rate of neural impulses into a muscle.)

Many people mistakenly assume that the designations of slow, intermediate, and fast refer to the speed of contraction of the classes of muscle fibers—or groups of muscle fibers, known as "motor units." In fact, what these designations indicate are the respective fatigue rates of these fibers: there are "slow-fatiguing," "intermediate-fatiguing," and "fast-fatiguing" fibers. Even though the force output from fast-twitch fibers is much greater than the force output from slow-twitch fibers, what you will observe on a molecular basis is that the twitch velocity of fast-twitch fibers is actually slower than it is with slow-twitch fibers. Moreover, not only is the twitch velocity slower in fast-twitch muscle fibers, but so is the rate of recovery. The more slowly a muscle fiber fatigues, the more quickly it recovers.

Looked at in this context, we note that slow-twitch fibers fatigue slowly but recover quickly; fast-twitch fibers (because their force output is so high, and because they burn through higher amounts of glycogen than slow-twitch fibers) fatigue quickly and recover slowly; while intermediate-twitch fibers fall somewhere in the middle of these two extremes in their recovery ability.

To understand why fast-twitch fibers produce more force, it is first necessary to understand something of the nature of how muscle fibers contract. This requires knowledge of the aforementioned motor unit.

THE MOTOR UNIT

A motor unit is a group of identical-twitch fibers (which, for our purposes, we'll again classify simplistically as fast-twitch, intermediate-twitch, and slow-twitch) serviced by one nerve that comes down into a muscle like an electrical cord. Off of this nerve, and spread throughout the width and breadth of the muscle, are appendages that resemble branches of a tree.

Each of these tipped branches (nerves) connects to a muscle fiber in a given motor unit of a similar twitch profile.

Let's investigate how this process works when the body is activating a slow-twitch motor unit. To begin, all of the slow-twitch muscle fibers at the ends of these tipped branches in this particular motor unit are going to be distributed evenly and homogeneously throughout the volume of a muscle. They are considered a "unit" even though they are separate from each other and spread all over the architecture of the muscle. The reason they are considered a unit is that they all track back through those same tipped branches to the same trunk of the tree, which, as we've seen, is a single motor nerve. Slow-twitch motor units are typically small, having approximately 100 fibers per unit.

Fast-twitch motor units have a similar composition in that they also have a tree trunk (or single motor nerve) coming down and also have "branches" spreading out from it, but they connect only to other fast-twitch fibers that are likewise distributed homogeneously throughout the volume of a given muscle. All of them, just as with the slow-twitch motor units, are attached via those branches back to the trunk or motor nerve. Compared with the slow-twitch motor units, fast-twitch motor units have a much larger number of muscle fibers that they embrace. So, instead of having a motor unit that is slow-twitch and has 100 fibers connected to it, a fast-twitch motor unit might have approximately 10,000 fibers connected to it. When you activate a motor unit, whether slow-twitch or fast-twitch, as the nerve impulse comes down the motor nerve and spreads out among its branches to hit all of the fibers in a particular motor unit, 100 percent of those involved fibers are going to contract with 100 percent of their force capability.

When a slow-twitch motor unit is activated, all 100 of its fibers contract simultaneously. (This is referred to as the "all or none" law of muscle physiology.) Likewise, when a fast-twitch motor unit is activated, all 10,000 of its fibers are going to contract simultaneously with 100 percent of their force. Since slow-twitch motor units take up less space in any given muscle, you're going to have a lot more slow-twitch motor units, per unit of muscle, than you do fast-twitch motor units, which means you're going to have a lot more "tree trunks" spreading out their 100 branches. Consequently, when slow-twitch motor units are triggered, you're going to be activating somewhere in the neighborhood of 1,000 of them. Fast-twitch motor units, by contrast, are much bigger (you have 10,000 fibers per motor unit), so that when you activate them, you're going to activate only 50 or 100 of these motor units, because each one of their motor units is so big.

SEQUENTIAL RECRUITMENT

Motor units can be contracted either simultaneously, such as when your muscles are made to contract against a very heavy load, or sequentially, such as when the activity you are performing involves a more modest load but is continued over a period during which certain lower-order fibers fatigue out and are replaced by a progressive recruitment of higher-order motor units. For example, sequential recruitment would occur during the course of a set of a resistance exercise, whereby you would perform a series of contractions and extensions (repetitions) over a time frame of, say, sixty to ninety seconds, until you are no longer capable of completing a contraction.

In such a scenario, you would be progressively fatiguing muscle fibers in order of motor-unit size and, therefore, in order of motor-unit type. You would first recruit your smallest motor units, which are the slow-twitch, and then move on to recruit the intermediate-twitch motor units, your next largest. If you fatigued those out, you would finally recruit your fast-twitch motor units. Although you're going to recruit fewer fast-twitch motor units, each one of these motor units is going to have 10,000 fibers being activated at once.

Time is an important factor in the recruitment process as well, in that as you fatigue through the slow-twitch motor units, you will proceed up to the next-largest motor units, the intermediate-twitch. If you fatigue through those quickly enough so that the slow- and intermediate-twitch motor units do not have time to recover, then (and only then) you proceed to recruit the fast-twitch motor units, thereby ensuring a sequential recruitment and fatiguing of all of the available motor units. This results in the most thorough involvement (and thus stimulation) of the muscle or muscle groups that you are training.

What determines the recruitment rate of the fibers within the muscles over a given unit of time is the load you have selected for your exercise. If you use a weight that is too light, the load will not be meaningful enough. You will recruit the slow-twitch fibers into service, but because they fatigue so slowly, by the time you have started to recruit the intermediate fibers, some of those same slow-twitch motor units will have started to recover. They will then be recycled back into the contraction process, thus preventing you from ever engaging the higher-order muscle fibers.

Conversely, if you select a weight that's too heavy, such as one that allows you to perform only one or two repetitions, you will recruit all of the available motor units—slow-twitch, intermediate-twitch, and fast-twitch—in tandem. What happens in this scenario is that as soon as your fast-twitch motor units fall out of the equation (because they're going to fatigue the quickest), you're not going to have enough force-producing ability left to perform a third repetition. Thus, the set will terminate before you've had the opportunity to thoroughly involve and stimulate the bulk of your slow- and intermediate-twitch fibers.

This is why it is desirable to employ a moderately heavy weight that allows you to progress through all three motor-unit types quickly enough to recruit them all, but not so quickly that only the fast-twitch fibers receive the bulk of the stimulation, and not so slowly that the slow- and/or intermediate-twitch motor units can recover and you end up cycling through the same lower-order motor units again. That would leave the bulk of the fibers in the muscle that you are training largely unstimulated.

RECOVERY OF FIBERS

Two different aspects of recovery need to be distinguished. One is the temporary recovery of the motor units—the slow-twitch, intermediate-twitch, and fast-twitch. The other is the recovery of the energy and resources that are expended during a workout. What we're referring to in this context is recovery of the motor units involved to the point where they are capable of contracting again. When the neural transmitter descends down the nerve and empties into the cleft between the nerve and the muscle cell to activate the muscle, only a brief period is required for that neural transmitter to be taken back up into the nerve, resynthesized, and made available for recruitment and contraction again.

To illustrate what's going on here, let's say you are performing a workout that requires you to leg-press 160 pounds. You are able to accomplish ten repetitions but fail to complete an eleventh. Should you attempt to perform a leg press exercise again before the fast-twitch fibers in your legs have had time to fully recover (and assuming the fast-twitch motor units were called into play, full recovery may not take place for weeks), when your body attempts to recruit those same fast-twitch fibers again, they will be unavailable.

The reason for this is that the fast-twitch motor units account for perhaps only the last two to twenty seconds of contraction. You would normally tap these fibers only in a true emergency situation, which, in hunter-gatherer times, would have occurred relatively infrequently. By their nature, these fibers, once tapped, can take four to ten days (or longer) to fully recover. Consequently, were you to return to the gym three days after your last workout and attempt to perform another set of leg presses, you would find that you are now hitting a point of momentary muscular failure two to three repetitions earlier than you did in your last workout. That's because the fast-twitch motor units would not be available for recruitment after three days of rest. Your slowest-twitch motor units, by contrast, would be available for recruitment again after a rest of ninety seconds.

This explains why people can exercise to a point of muscular failure on a set of leg presses and, immediately upon concluding the set, find that they lack the strength to stand up, but after a brief rest of only thirty seconds to a minute, they can stand up, walk out of the gym, and drive home without a problem. Ninety seconds of respite, then, is sufficient time to allow for recovery of the lower-order fibers, but the faster-twitch fibers are still several days away from being fully recovered and thus incapable of being recruited again before that time has elapsed.

Exercise, in keeping with our medicine analogy, is a potent stimulus that acts on an organism—your body, in this instance—and causes it to produce an adaptive response, providing that you allow it the time it requires to accomplish this objective. Understanding this, you can see that in order for progress to continue, you have to raise the stimulus/intensity of the exercise to which you are exposing your body.

Now let's say that rather than selecting resistance training as your mode of exercise, you have opted for walking. This being the case, in order to raise the stimulus/intensity of this mode of physical activity, over time, you will have to transition from walking, to fast walking, to jogging. Then, if you want to raise the stimulus/intensity high enough to tap into those faster-twitch motor units and really stimulate all of the fibers in your leg muscles, you will have to ultimately transition from jogging to sprinting. Keep in mind that if we're going to use this modality of exercise to accomplish our goals, at every level that we choose to increase the intensity to meet those goals, we will be exponentially increasing the amount of force that our bodies encounter and, therefore, increasing the amount of risk to which we are subjecting our bodies in terms of damage—both short-term and long-term.

Since we *do* have a choice as to what form of exercise we can employ, we don't have to undermine our health in the process of attempting to enhance our fitness. This is where strength training comes to the fore as a superior modality. For one thing, with proper resistance training, we are going to be using movements that correctly correspond with (or track) muscle and joint function. Therefore, we're not going to be placing any joints or musculature in a vulnerable position that, as we increase the stimulus/intensity, will put us at significant risk for injury.

Second, we will employ a protocol that, rather than recruiting fast-twitch fibers in tandem with the slow- and intermediate-twitch fibers (as occurs with activities such as sprinting), we will recruit motor units in a systematic, orderly fashion. First we will recruit and fatigue the slow-twitch motor units, but we will be recruiting these quickly enough that they cannot recover during the course of our exercise. That means that we also are going to be recruiting and fatiguing the intermediate-twitch and then, in sequential fashion, the fast-twitch motor units—as opposed to recruiting them simultaneously. And while our muscles are recruiting and fatiguing motor units in an orderly recruitment pattern, motor units are falling out because of fatigue.

The effect is that we are actually becoming weaker during the set, so that we are at our weakest at the point where we finally recruit those fast-twitch motor units. With strength training, we are using a stimulus that allows us to get at those fast-twitch motor units, but by the time we recruit them, we will have fatigued ourselves so deeply that we are literally "too weak" to bring harm to ourselves.

Strength training is the only modality in which you can bring a potent stimulus for positive change to the body and as you raise the stimulus/intensity level, you are actually becoming weaker and, therefore, inflicting less force on your body. This is one of the unique advantages of strength training. The forces are low to begin with: if you start with a weight of 100 pounds, it stays at 100 pounds, requiring the same amount of force to move it at the end of the set as it does at the beginning, even as your fiber recruitment and rate of fatigue increase.

It should be pointed out that all injuries are caused by muscular or mechanical structures encountering forces that exceed their strength, and this doesn't happen with proper strength training. Force is defined as mass $\times$ acceleration. Acceleration is a factor that can be increased exponentially, which can be dangerous. There are plenty of ways to recruit fast-twitch motor units, but there are very few ways in which to do so safely. For instance, fast-twitch motor units can be engaged by performing sprints or in exercise modalities such as plyometrics, which involve jumping off of boxes. When you recruit fast-twitch motor units by performing such activities, you are recruiting them in tandem with the slow- and intermediate-twitch motor units. The same situation occurs when you attempt a single lift of a heavy weight, such as in power lifting.

This situation has the potential to cause two bad outcomes. For starters, it allows you to produce an amount of force with your musculature that could well exceed your body's structural capability. If that's not deterrent enough, you're going to be unable to continue as soon as the fastest-twitch motor units fall out, with the result that when you reach that level of fatigue, you have still not significantly fatigued your lower-order motor units and thus have missed out on two-thirds of the productive capability of an exercise.

Proper strength training does exactly the opposite. Rather than recruiting all muscle fibers in tandem, it recruits them in a sequential, orderly fashion and taps the fast-twitch motor units last, *after* you've tapped out all of the other, lower-order fibers. This yields a far more thorough stimulation of your musculature and of your metabolism. There isn't a rock that's left unturned. Not only are all fiber types stimulated, but also, because of the tie-in of the metabolic pathways to mechanical movement, you're involving everything related to fitness in the organism by using this protocol.

THE DOSAGE: ONE SET TO FAILURE

Having determined the ingredients of the necessary medicine, it remains to determine how much of it we require at any one interval—that is, its dosage. While many exercise authorities claim that multiple sets of a particular exercise should be performed (typically, three sets of ten repetitions), the scientific literature suggests that one set performed in the manner that we advocate is all the stimulus that is required.

In 1997, physiologists conducted a ten-week training study of recreational weight lifters in which various set schemes were tested. They concluded that one set per exercise was just as effective as two and four sets for improving muscular size, strength, and upper-body power.[2] In addition, physiologists R. N. Carpinelli and R. M. Otto conducted a study out of Adelphi University that surveyed all of the known scientific literature concerning single-set versus multiple-set resistance training. They found that, on the whole, performing multiple sets brought absolutely *no* additional increase in results compared with single-set training. The literature came down overwhelmingly in favor of a single set of exercise as being sufficient; only two out of the forty-seven studies surveyed showed any benefit (and a marginal improvement at that) to be had from the performance of multiple sets.[3]

Other studies support this conclusion. For instance, researchers examining strength gains in seventy-seven subjects who performed one, two, or three sets of upper-body exercise over a ten-week training period established that all three exercise groups made similar improvements in upper-body muscle strength.[4] Yet another study, this one comparing strength gains in thirty-eight subjects who performed one or three sets of lower-body exercise over a fourteen-week period, documented similar improvements in lower-body strength, with an increase in knee flexion and knee extension strength of roughly 15 percent.[5]

A further study published in the journal *Medicine and Science in Sports and Exercise* also established that one set of high-intensity resistance training was just as effective as three sets for increasing knee extension and knee flexion isometric torque as well as muscle thickness in previously untrained adults.[6]

The bottom line is that a single set taken to a point of positive failure is a sufficient stimulus to trigger the growth and strength mechanism of the body into motion. Additional sets produce nothing but more time spent in the gym.

EXERCISE IN ACCORD WITH MUSCLE AND JOINT FUNCTION

Proper exercise tracks muscle and joint function perfectly. The shoulder muscles, for instance, can draw the arms forward, backward, or out to the sides. Proper resistance exercise for the lateral head of this muscle group allows the muscles to perform their function against resistance— whether provided by a machine or with free weights.

We've touched on the fact that, ideally, exercise should be performed in accord with muscle and joint function, so that one can stimulate one's muscles efficiently and sufficiently in a manner that does not bring excess force to the body. In contrast are the various "cross-training" programs that are commonplace in most commercial gymnasiums, wherein clients climb ropes, drag weighted sleds, throw medicine balls, and so forth.

These programs certainly require high levels of exertion, and engaging in them will produce some elements of fatigue, along with some weakening of muscles and some metabolic effect on

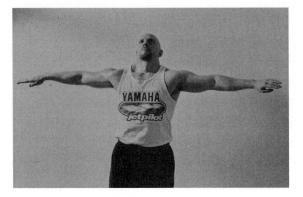
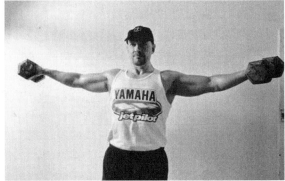

the systems of the body, but such activities are not typically performed in accordance with muscle and joint function. As a result, while these activities can cause you to produce a lot of metabolic work and a lot of metabolic by-products of fatigue, you will not necessarily be achieving efficient muscular loading and recruitment of motor units, accompanied by the subsequent weakening of the targeted muscles. Therefore, they are not a particularly potent stimulus for positive adaptation or growth. Moreover, you are also accumulating huge amounts of force in the process of their performance, which can lead to injuries to your joints and connective tissues—most notably, your knees and your back—and put you on the path to the development of arthritis.

A key problem with such eclectic training approaches is that the training effect from the activity is dissipated. To follow through with our analogy, it would be tantamount to a diluted concentration of one's medicine. You will end up wasting a lot of metabolic energy exerting yourself in an activity that is nonproductive in terms of its potential stimulus for adaptation. Your body would much rather have five muscle groups contributing 20 percent of their energy capacity to an activity than have any one muscle group contributing 100 percent, so you are playing into the conservation-of-energy preference of your genome. Whereas the former energy expenditure is over with the completion of the activity, the latter requires ongoing energy to produce the adaptive response you desire, such as more muscle tissue; thus, its energy cost is, in the long run, far greater to the organism. Remember that the body is loathe to expend energy, particularly when stimulated to expend more of it with the production of more muscle tissue, and it will avoid doing so whenever possible.

One reason the authors' facilities have been successful in producing substantial fitness and health benefits for clients is that we actually *know* what the required stimulus is—and we know that it isn't merely physical activity. We recognize that it's activity performed at a threshold level of intensity that recruits all of the available motor units in a sequential fashion within a given time frame to ensure thorough muscle fiber involvement and fatiguing.

We further recognize that the stimulus is to some extent multifactorial, but all of these factors are related to the stimulus/intensity being high. If the stimulus/intensity is high, you are going to tap all three classifications of motor units; you're going to produce a high level of what we refer to as "inroad"—or momentary fatiguing or weakening of the muscle. You will be training with a meaningful load and using a heavy enough weight to induce a mechanical stress on the musculature, which is one of the components of the stimulus. As you move from slow- to intermediate- to fast-twitch motor units in your recruitment pattern, your metabolism will shift toward an anaerobic nature, which results in the metabolism of glucose at a rate that allows for the accumulation of lactic acid and other by-products of fatigue. This condition also appears to be beneficial to the stimulus process.

Yes, we could accomplish this result to some extent by putting a car in neutral and having you push it around, but we can do it better by having a knowledge of muscle and joint function and actually using that to our advantage. It is the job of an informed and responsible trainer to make you strong up to and beyond the age of forty-seven (the time when your genome says you should have been dead). If we were to choose alternate forms of exercise, you might well accumulate too much wear and tear in the process of exercising and end up crippled by the time you reached the age of fifty.

TIME AS A FACTOR IN OPTIMAL STIMULATION

For exercise to be optimal, as many muscle fibers as possible must be called into play and fatigued. Moreover, that fatigue has to occur quickly enough so that you're not giving your quickest-recovering motor units time to recover and kick back into play, which would spare the recruitment of your fastest-twitch motor units. Consequently, depending on the protocol you are using, as well as the cadence with which you are lifting the resistance (which we'll get to shortly), the fatigue rate should fall anywhere between forty seconds and two and a half minutes. Optimally, we're looking at forty-five to ninety seconds for a particular set of exercise as the desired time frame for reaching a maximum level of fatigue. This will ensure an orderly recruitment of all the different muscle fibers and also ensure that you will be tapping the fast-twitch motor units that possess the most glycogen.

DOSING FREQUENCY: HOW OFTEN YOU SHOULD EXERCISE

Having established the appropriate medicine and the appropriate dose, we now need to determine an optimal dosing frequency. We've noted that the stimulus of exercise yields the potential to do one of two things: it can stimulate positive change, or it can interfere with the adaptation process if the stimulus is brought back to the body before the adaptation process has been completed. (See Figure 3.1.)

It might be said metaphorically that every time you work out, you are digging a hole, or making an inroad, in your energy reserves. This catabolic state of breaking down and weakening must be balanced by an anabolic state of recovery and building up. So, if you can be said to be digging a hole when you apply the exercise stimulus to your muscles, then you have to allow enough time for that hole to be filled back up (the recovery process), and you also have to allow enough time for some additional material to be piled on top of that hole (overcompensation) to bring it up to a level higher than it was before. If you start digging again before the hole is refilled, you don't make the mound bigger; you instead dig a deeper and deeper hole. How often you should dig is analogous to how often you should work out. (See Figure 3.2.)

Obviously, you should not work out before recovery and full adaptation from the previous workout takes place—but how long is this, on average? We can share with you the average length of time that we have found to be most beneficial based on our own thirty-plus years of training, in addition to our experience in supervising in excess of 150,000 workouts and performing informal studies on the subject. Perhaps more significantly, we can also share with you the findings of exercise physiology studies regarding what happens as a result of a high-intensity workout stimulus being applied to the muscles and how long the recovery and overcompensation process typically takes.

According to the medical literature, the more intensely the muscles are made to contract, the more damage or microtrauma takes place at a cellular level.[7] Consequently, the greater the intensity of the workout, the more time must be allowed for the repair and growth of the tissue that was stimulated by the workout. It is this process of repair that makes the muscle fibers bigger and stronger.[8]

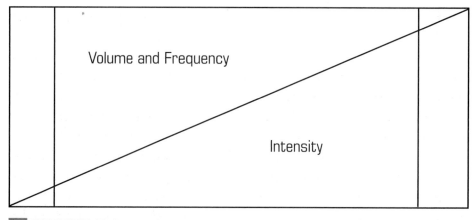

■ FIGURE 3.1.

For exercise to be time efficient, it must be of a high intensity. As the intensity of your exercise increases, you must reduce both the volume and frequency. Exercise of long duration or high frequency is possible only with low-intensity activity. From a biologic standpoint, you want to provide a stimulus that will cause your body to adapt favorably.

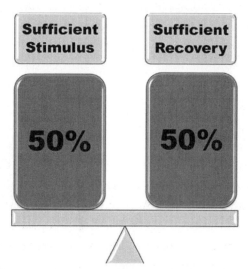

■ FIGURE 3.2.

You must allow the body time to replenish the resources that were consumed. If you bring the inroading stimulus back to your body before it has completed the adaptive response, you will interfere with the response. Providing a sufficiently intense stimulus is 50 percent of the adaptation equation, with sufficient recovery being the other 50 percent. This is why you must limit yourself to one workout per week.

The workout itself causes some degree of temporary damage to the muscle fibers, the majority of which results from the lowering of the resistance (the negative, or eccentric, portion of the contraction), as opposed to the raising of it.[9] In the twenty-four hours that follow a workout, inflammation sets in, during which white blood cells (neutrophils) are increased and are mobilized to the site of the injury.[10] It is during those first twenty-four hours that lysosomes—enzymes that break down and metabolize damaged tissue—are produced, which adds to the inflammatory process.[11] For the next several days, additional cells (macrophages) that assist in synthesizing other chemicals in response to inflammation aid in the accumulation of lysosomes. One of these is PGE2, a chemical that is believed to make nerves within muscles more sensitive to pain. This process explains to some degree the perception of soreness that typically follows twenty-four to thirty-six hours after a workout and can, in some instances, last a week or more.[12] This inflammatory response brings further damage to the muscles and can continue for several days after the workout.[13]

After these inflammation responses have been completed, signs of tissue remodeling, or building of muscle, are then observed.[14] The muscle fibers build back to their preworkout size and then, if further time is allowed, will build up to a level that is greater than it was before the workout. The length of time required for the entire process to complete itself is dependent on the intensity of the workout stimulus and the corresponding damage to the muscle fibers.[15] Typically, it falls in the neighborhood of five days (on the quick side of things) to six weeks.[16]

While the preceding summary reflects a microscopic view of what happens as a result of exercise, other studies, as previously mentioned, have looked at training frequency macroscopically, examining the effects of training different groups of people (from senior citizens to younger subjects) with one, two, or more workouts per week. All of these studies have also come to the conclusion that training once a week produces all of the benefits to be had from a workout program and that training more frequently serves no additional purpose.[17] Further verification for training once a week came from a study conducted by Utah State University's Strength Laboratory that was designed specifically to compare the effects of performing a single set of leg presses, with one group performing the exercise once a week and a second group performing it twice a week. At the end of the study, the experimenters concluded that "performing a single set of leg presses once or twice a week results in statistically similar strength gains."[18]

Some people might be inclined to think that once-a-week training is sufficient only for males, who typically are bigger and stronger than females and thus produce a deeper inroading stimulus and greater accumulated by-products of fatigue, which would naturally take longer for the body to process than would a lesser amount of accumulated by-products of fatigue. However, the Utah State study consisted entirely of female subjects, establishing that once-a-week training is sufficient for both sexes.

As enlightening as this study is, it should be pointed out that its duration was only eight weeks. We believe, based on our experience, that had the study been protracted out to ten or twelve weeks, the researchers would have noted evidence of a strongly negative effect among the subjects who were made to perform a second weekly workout. In fact, in our opinion, most of the studies that have been conducted on strength training thus far have not been carried out long enough to detect the "downside" of which we have become aware as personal trainers.

This particular study suggests that whether you train once or twice a week, you net out the same—which may well be true with beginning subjects over an eight-week time span (and which argues against performing 100 percent more exercise for zero percent additional return on your time and effort investment). Nevertheless, even at best, the data suggest that if you train twice a week, the second workout isn't doing anything positive and serves only to waste your time. The reality is that by week twelve, had the study been carried out that long, you would have noted that not only were you wasting your time by performing a second weekly workout, but also you were actually starting to regress and would be unable to lift the same amount of weight for the same time-under-load (or repetition) ranges.

This phenomenon was established clinically in a pair of studies that were conducted eight years apart. In these controlled experiments, the researchers examined the rate of progress of two groups of subjects—one group training three days a week and the other group training two days a week. The experimenters then reduced the frequency of the training, cutting back the group that was training three times a week to twice a week, and cutting back the group that was training two times a week to once a week. The experimenters noted that the subjects' rate of progress—measured on an absolute basis per unit of time—improved markedly.[19]

Similar results have been reported in other studies involving subjects of varying ages, wherein the experimenters decreased the subjects' training frequency and found that workout performances improved substantially. In one study involving senior citizens, conducted by the Academic Health Care Center of the New York College of Osteopathic Medicine in conjunction with the Department of Physical Therapy at the New York Institute of Technology's School of Health Professions, in Old Westbury, New York, the results of seniors who exercised once a week were compared against a group of seniors who trained twice a week. The researchers found "no difference in strength changes between training once a week versus twice a week after 9 weeks." They added, "One set of exercises performed once weekly to muscle fatigue improved strength as well as twice a week in the older adult."[20]

A Trainer's Input

I have been training people on a one-to-one basis since I was eighteen years old. I've long understood that continued results from exercise are dependent on the proper manipulation of stimulus and recovery. This became clinically obvious to me while I was attending the University of New Orleans as an undergraduate in exercise physiology while at the same time training clients at a local Nautilus club using high-intensity training methods. As I had already been training clients for several years, I often used the data collected from my clientele for class papers and projects. One of my goals during this period was to determine the approximate amount of time (years) it took most clients to approach their maximum genetic potential for strength. As it turned out, most subjects approached this limit in approximately two years, as long as the stimulus (S) and recovery (R) variables were properly balanced.

However, during the original data analysis, several other issues became apparent. If the equation was not balanced (S ≠ R), subjects hit an artificial plateau. This was evident when data were culled and contrasted from client workouts that varied in frequency from once to twice a week and also from workouts that contrasted the results of clients who supplemented one workout per week with additional activities, which generally took the form of some type of endurance training. Figure 3.3 indicates this phenomenon.

As you can see, the general pattern reveals that most clients showed greater initial progress (i.e., strength increases) on a twice-per-week training schedule versus once-per-week, but they hit a plateau much sooner. While clients who trained once per week did not initially gain as quickly as those who trained twice per week, their rate of improvement was comparable—and then the difference became marked, as their progress never flatlined; they continued to improve for a much *longer* period than did the twice-a-week group.

The "linear adaptation" line is fictional, indicating the belief of many laypeople that progress to one's genetic potential is a direct, or linear, process rather than a curvilinear one. As you can see from contrasting this line with the other two lines, that isn't the way it works in reality. In fact, when a particular twice-per-week subject reduced his or her frequency of training to once per week, strength increases were almost immediate and continuous. From my recollection, this occurred in approximately 97 percent of the original subjects tested. Rarely did the reverse occur, although a small percentage of subjects progressed less when transitioning to the once-per-week schedule. However small the number was (3 percent), I could not ignore this statistic and have spent my ensuing career as a trainer researching and attempting to understand this interindividual variability in response to resistance exercise. [Authors' note: Much of the research in Chapter 8 is the result of Ryan Hall's labor in addressing the genetic components that affect issues such as training volume and frequency.] I know that most of us practicing high-intensity training have had similar experiences with regard to training clients, with the vast majority of clients responding best (and for longer periods) with a once-a-week protocol.

**—Ryan Hall, Personal Trainer, One to One Personal Training
and Clinical Exercise, LLC, New Orleans**

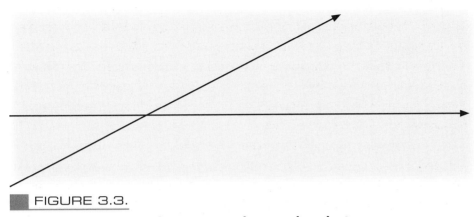

FIGURE 3.3.

Results of once-a-week workouts versus twice-a-week workouts.

A BIOLOGIC MODEL

The process of growing new muscle can be likened to the process of growing new skin after a burn or a cut. The injury is a stimulus to engage the body's growth and repair mechanism to heal and repair damaged tissue. The next time you sustain an injury of this type, observe how long it takes your body to produce this new tissue. Typically, it's as much as a week to two weeks—and that's to produce a lot *less* tissue than what a proper training stimulus has been shown to prompt the body to produce (0.66 to 1.1 pounds).

So, if you've applied a more potent stimulus to prompt your body to produce a lot more tissue, it will take more time for your body to do so. Building muscle is actually a much slower process than healing a wound from a burn. A burn wound heals from the ectodermal germ line, where the healing rate is relatively faster, because epithelial cells turn over quickly. If you scratch your cornea, for instance, it's generally going to be healed in eight to twelve hours. Muscle tissue, in contrast, heals from the mesodermal germ line, where the healing rate is typically significantly slower. All in all—when you separate all the emotion and the positive feedback that many people derive from the training experience—solid biologic data indicate that an optimal training frequency for the vast majority of the population is no more than once a week.

The Big-Five Workout

The workout program in this chapter represents an ideal starting point, as well as a foundation to which you can return from time to time should you eventually decide to experiment with various tweaking protocols. If you do choose to deviate from this program later in your training to employ some of the protocols presented later in the book, it is important to return to this workout to assess your progress. Doing so will not only help you accurately measure your performance but also provide an effective way to stimulate the most muscle. The program has broad applicability to the population as a whole for achieving the most improvement and adaptation from exercise.

THE MUTUAL FUND OF EXERCISES

You can think of this workout as comparable to an initial financial investment. In the world of investment, participants who have historically realized the best performance are those who have purchased mutual funds. In contrast, investors who tend to buy and sell, continually changing their portfolios, typically magnify their losses. Even if the odd one occasionally hits it big, it is hard to isolate why a particular strategy worked (recall the "black swan" factor from the Introduction), and on average, this type of investor does not do as well as those who buy and hold a solid mutual fund.

Of the many mutual funds available, an index fund that tracks the total market, such as an S&P 500 index fund, will typically outperform 85 to 95 percent of all other mutual funds. This is true because the fund automatically buys only the five hundred stocks in the index. There is relatively little variation as a result of buying and selling new stocks and relatively little expense incurred in paying market analysts and fund managers. An even better example is a "Dow Five" fund that buys only the five best-valued stocks of the Dow industrials' ten top-performing stocks. So, if you have saved your first block of cash to invest and don't want to waste it on a bad offering, a good place to start would be with a reputable mutual fund.

A good workout program that does not change over time can be considered a reliable "index fund" of workouts. The program laid out here is based on the recovery-system characteristics of 85 to 95 percent of the population, in addition to data collected from supervising more than 150,000 workouts at both of the authors' facilities, involving training people one on one throughout the past eleven years.

As with investing, the newcomer to strength training is not at a point where it makes sense to consider some derivative hedge fund for his or her first deposit. Again, the wiser course is to choose an index fund that tracks the S&P 500 and to stay with that. Over time, even the most sophisticated money managers are going to underperform something that's generic and basic, and the same holds with protocols in exercise.

Our purpose is to give you a program that will have broad applicability and impart a lot of bang for your metabolic buck. It is not intended as an "ultimate bodybuilding routine" for someone who plans to enter a national competition, although this workout program may prove to be superior for that purpose as well. Psychologically, however, those who wish to go that route will want to be in a gym far more frequently than what we recommend, solely to soothe their training angst. Since we are not catering to that crowd, but rather focusing in on what the the human body requires to stimulate all of the metabolic benefits necessary to optimize human health and fitness, we have kept this training program as simple as possible.

EQUIPMENT

Before getting under way with the movements, it is beneficial to address the type of equipment to use—if a choice exists. A comprehensive campaign initiated by the manufacturers of free weights (which also tend to own the majority of bodybuilding and fitness publications) has been in progress since the late 1970s and has many people believing that free weights are much better than machines. The fact of the matter is that your muscles deal only with force-production requirements, which, in turn, are determined by the resistance to which the muscles are exposed—whether that resistance comes in the form of a free weight, a Nautilus machine, or a bucket of rocks. The scientific literature backs this up: according to the few properly performed studies that measured the effects of free weights versus machines, both are equally effective.[1]

Given the parity among virtually all forms of resistance training in their ability to stimulate muscle tissue to grow bigger and stronger, as well as the goal of training to a point where you can no longer produce enough force to lift the resistance, we advocate the use of machines for this purpose. No one wants to risk being pinned under a barbell at the point of muscular failure on free-weight exercises such as the bench press or squat. Since machines are safer and are at least as efficient as free weights at stimulating muscles, we see no upside to taking a risk that isn't required.

Of the scores of exercise machines available, we favor brands such as Nautilus and MedX, which are known to feature correct cam profiles that vary the resistance in accord with the strength curves of the muscles being trained. For proper training, the facility should have a minimum of five machines that can target the major muscle groups of the body.

The main reason we have a favorable inclination toward Nautilus machines, with a particular prejudice for the older generation (circa 1970–85), is that this equipment was the product of decades of research by an individual with a wide knowledge of muscle physiology. Considerable time, thought, effort, and money went into the design of these machines, and a lot more money went into research with the machines once they were created. Therefore, we know within one to two points exactly what kind of results can be expected from training with this type of equipment.

When Nautilus first came on the scene, only Universal and Marcy were making multistation resistance-training machines, along with, of course, free weights—barbells and dumbbells. Other equipment brands that came afterward are largely copies of Nautilus, made by people who simply wanted to get into the exercise equipment marketplace, rather than to "build a better mousetrap." It took almost forty years of testing and prototyping to develop the first Nautilus machine, and we flat-out don't see any other equipment manufacturers putting that same degree of thought and time into their designs.

Nautilus and Arthur Jones

Arthur Jones, the man who created Nautilus equipment, was among the first to devise effective equipment for dealing with the fact that muscles have differing levels of strength throughout their range of motion. These variations are a function of the muscles' physical relation to the bone, which moves and is always changing.

This strength curve can actually be measured at each point in a muscle's range of motion. In a barbell curl, for example, one might discover that the strength curve of the biceps muscle measures 10 pounds of force when the arm is perfectly straight, 25 pounds of force when the arm is bent 45 degrees, 39 pounds of force when the forearm is bent 90 degrees, 21 pounds of force when another 45 degrees of movement has occurred, and finally, when the hand is at the shoulder, perhaps 12 pounds of force can be produced. If these figures were plotted on a graph, the strength curve for the biceps would reveal that this muscle produces more or less force as the limb the muscle travels throughout the arc of its range of motion.

In that every muscle has its own strength curve, each one is different. The biceps, for instance, display a strength curve of weak-strong-weak as they contract, whereas the hamstrings display a strength curve of strong-weaker-weakest. If a round pulley is employed in the training of these muscles, such as with cable exercises and certain brands of machines, the trainee experiences a heavy start and a light finish—irrespective of the muscle group being trained. While this effect might well be fine for training a muscle group such as the hamstrings, it is completely mismatched for muscles such as the biceps and pectorals.

Since your muscles' strength changes during contraction, proper strength training must take this factor into account and thus requires a synchronous (or matched) loading (and deloading) of the musculature. That being the case, an even less effective approach is to be had with free weights. If, to follow up on the preceding example, you can produce only 10 pounds of force at the start of a set of barbell curls, but we give you a 35-pound barbell, you won't have the strength to move it—even though you would have the strength (and then some) to contract against this weight if you could bend it to the point of 90 degrees. So, since you can't even start the movement with 35 pounds, you instead select a 10-pound barbell, because you can move that weight. However, 10 pounds provides no effective overload at 45 degrees or 90 degrees of flexion and thus compromises the effectiveness of the training stimulus for producing a strength increase.

This is where Jones's offset cam represents a huge contribution to exercise science. Because the moment arm (the distance from the axis of rotation to the resistance) changes during a muscle's range of motion, the force required from a muscle to move even a 35-pound load can be tremendously divergent. If the moment arm is two inches, for example, then the inch pounds would be 70 (the work done 35 pounds $\times$ 2 inches = 70 pounds); if the moment arm is six inches, the inch pounds of force required to move the load would grow to 210; if the moment arm is ten inches, the inch pounds would be 350; and if the moment arm is zero, the inch pounds would also be zero.

The radius of a Nautilus cam varies the resistance (and hence the effective inch or foot pounds) as much or as little as necessary, adapting the resistance to those changing strength curves of human muscle in a manner that perfectly tracks their peaks and valleys. Thanks to Jones's efforts, not only was muscle able to be trained far more efficiently and thoroughly, but also muscular wear and tear was notably reduced. The Nautilus cam

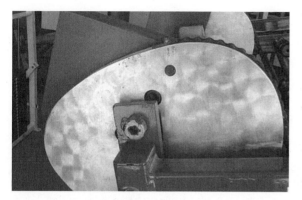

The radius of the Nautilus cam is smaller during the start position of the biceps curl.

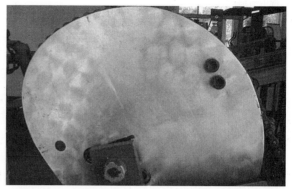

The radius of the cam increases as the muscle contracts, thereby increasing the resistance of the machine to track properly with the increasing strength of the biceps.

allowed the muscles to be exposed to a full range of resistance in balance with their actual force output.

Jones then patented his cams, which meant that competing equipment manufacturers could not simply copy them; they had to produce *different* ones. Consequently, since the strength curves of his cams were correct, the others were to a large extent incorrect. Jones once referred to his equipment as being "machines without compromise"—and his original machines reflected this claim. For all of these reasons, Nautilus machines receive a bold checkmark from both of us as being preferred equipment for workouts, particularly the older machines, which were designed under his stewardship. Similarly, we recommend any of the machines made by MedX that Jones had a hand in developing, because the same degree of effort and research went into their design.

Equipment Basics

We describe these exercises as they should be performed on Nautilus or MedX equipment, which we hold to be the best exercise machines on the market. As noted, this is owing to the accuracy of their cam profiles and their design features, which accurately track muscle and joint function. We strongly recommend that, wherever possible, you use these brands of

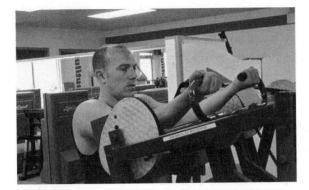
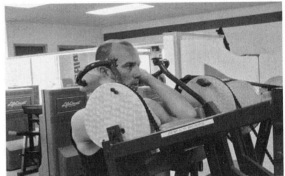

When a trainee trains his biceps on a Nautilus multi biceps machine, the radius of the cam is in perfect sync with the trainee's biceps muscles: smaller when he is weaker and bigger when he is stronger.

equipment. That said, other equipment manufacturers such as Hammer Strength and Southern Xercise Inc. also offer excellent machines that are, for the most part, biomechanically correct and will effectively and safely stimulate the muscles of the legs and upper body.

As for what machines a trainee should look for in a good gym, we recommend a facility that has the pieces that will allow a workout consisting of the exercises featured in this chapter: pulldown, leg press, seated row, chest press, and overhead press. In a broader sense, we want you to avail yourself of equipment that has been engineered to accurately address not only biomechanical and alignment functions but also the dimensions of strength curve. It's important to match the applied resistance to a muscle's force output at a particular point of the range of motion based on joint angle, because the goal is to reach a state of positive muscular failure as a result of deeply inroading the musculature in a prescribed period. You want to ensure that muscular failure has occurred because as complete as possible a level of fatigue has been reached, rather than as a result of a mechanical mismatch between the equipment's strength curve and the strength curve of the body's muscles.

This is not to suggest that if you train in a commercial gym that has alternative equipment choices, you won't be able to have a productive workout. The same principles will apply: you should employ the same time-under-load signatures (as explained later in the chapter) and as many reps as you can perform in strict form. If this isn't possible, consider purchasing a power rack and an Olympic barbell set and training at home. You can perform the Big-Five exercises on basic equipment pretty easily, and a power rack will provide a large measure of safety in that it will prevent you from being pinned underneath a barbell when you reach muscular failure.

THE BIG FIVE

This program consists exclusively of compound exercises—those that involve rotation around several joint axes—and thus involve several muscle groups per exercise. A "core" of three exercises will work all of the major muscular structures of the body. Called the Big Three, they are the leg press, pulldown, and chest press. Added to this core are an overhead press and a seated (or compound) row, to create the Big Five. These exercises are big but simple movements that involve multiple muscle groups and are also easy for the average person to coordinate and perform. Instead of devoting a large portion of your attention and mental intensity to the coordination of a complex movement, you perform a movement that is simple and natural, so the majority of your intensity and focus can be placed on performing hard work rather than on trying to execute two opposing actions.

Later sections in the chapter will explain how to perform the repetitions and record progress. Now, though, let's run through the details of each of the exercises.

Seated Row

The first exercise is a seated row, popularly referred to as an upper-body "pulling" exercise. It targets the torso musculature on the posterior aspect of the torso (the back) and, as a consequence, also involves the muscles that flex the upper extremity.

Muscle Structures Involved. The seated row involves the latissimus dorsi muscles, the rhomboid musculature (which is located between the shoulder blades and serves to draw them together), and the spinal extensor muscles, running from the base of your sacrum to the back of your head. Those will be involved as a secondary component, along with all the muscles of the

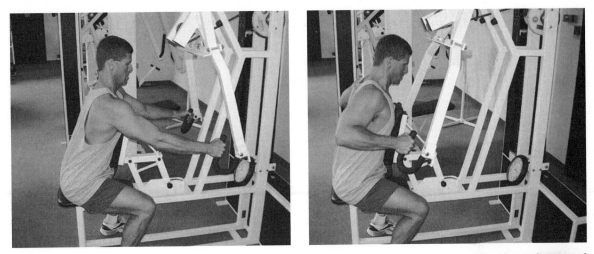

Seated row (start and finish position)

flexor side of the forearm that flex your wrist and the biceps and brachio-radilas muscles that bend your arm at the elbow joint.

Exercise Performance. When you're performing the seated row, the position of your arms is going to be predicated somewhat on the position of the handgrips of the machine relative to your shoulder width. Ideally, this should be a "natural" position: you should not be trying to tuck your elbows in or flare them out; rather, let them ride neutrally in the natural plane along which they tend to want to move—tracking in line with your hands, wrists, and shoulders.

Chest Press

After the seated row, your next exercise will be the chest press. The chest press falls into the category of upper-body "pushing" exercise, which involves the muscles on the anterior aspect (or front) of the torso that, when engaged, serve to move resistance away from the body.

Muscle Structures Involved. The chest press involves the triceps muscles on the back of the upper arm to a great extent, in addition to the deltoid musculature surrounding the shoulder joint. The pectoral muscles (chest

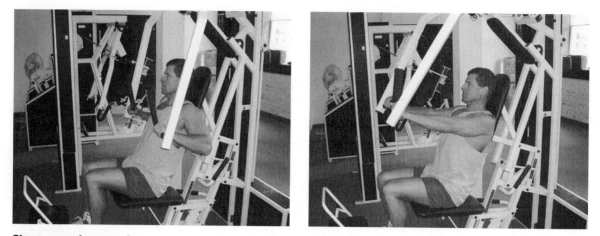

Chest press (start and finish position)

muscles), both pectoralis major and pectoralis minor, are also strongly stimulated by the performance of this exercise.

Exercise Performance. When performing the chest press, you will be pushing the handles of the machine away from your body while simultaneously pulling the humerus toward the midline of your body as your arms extend. Start the movement with the plane of your palms at the anterior axillary line (or the front) of the armpit. (It isn't necessary or desirable to attempt to increase your range of motion by driving your arms back behind you as far as possible, because that will overstretch the shoulder capsule and place needless tension on the biceps tendon at the humeral head.) It is important that you neither tuck nor flare your arms excessively; they should be kept at a 45-degree angle if you're holding the handles appropriately to start.

Now press your arms forward smoothly, and stop just short of lockout, so that the muscle stays loaded and you're not resting on a bone-on-bone tower with your elbows locked. When you're lowering the weight, the lower turnaround should be performed when your palms are about even with the front portion of your chest. (Often we will not let our clients bring the plane of the humerus much beyond the plane of the midtorso in a backward direction, so that their elbows are not going to get pinned back behind them.) In other words, bring your elbows back only slightly farther than they would be if you were performing the exercise while lying on the floor with a barbell.

Concentrate on keeping your shoulders tucked down as you perform this exercise. One way of ensuring that you do is to first shrug as high as you can toward your ears, and then have your trainer place his or her hands underneath your elbows while you press them down. This act of drawing your shoulders down is the position in which you want to keep your shoulders while you're performing the chest press. If you aren't aware of this position, what will happen is that as you weaken during the course of the set, the exercise becomes harder to perform. As fatigue starts to set in, many clients will start to draw their arms into a tuck position and shrug their shoulders up in an attempt to transfer the load off their pectoralis musculature and onto their trapezius musculature.

Even among champion bodybuilders working out, it is not uncommon to observe that as the exercise becomes progressively harder to perform, they tuck their shoulders up toward their ears as a natural reflex to recruit the trapezius muscle to complete the movement. This tendency is one of the reasons that some people develop pain in the center of the back, between the shoulder blades, when they perform chest presses of both the vertical and horizontal varieties, as they end up activating their rhomboid muscles to draw their shoulder blades together so that they can then activate the trapezius to try to bear the weight.

Also, we don't advocate performing incline or decline presses if a trainee is already performing a chest press. Some trainees who want to develop a thick "upper chest" believe that incline work is the best way to stress this region of the pectoral muscles. Their mistake is confusing the pec minor with the upper pec. A lot of trainees are of the mind-set that the upper region of the pectoral muscle is the "pec minor" muscle, when in reality what they are referring to is the clavicular portion of the pectoralis major muscle. The pectoralis minor sits underneath the pectoralis major and attaches to the ribs at several different levels, coming up and into the upper humerus at the level of the glenoid. The pectoralis minor contributes to the adduction of your humerus as your upper arm extends. So, both the pectoralis minor and the pectoralis major are already strongly activated in the performance of the chest press.

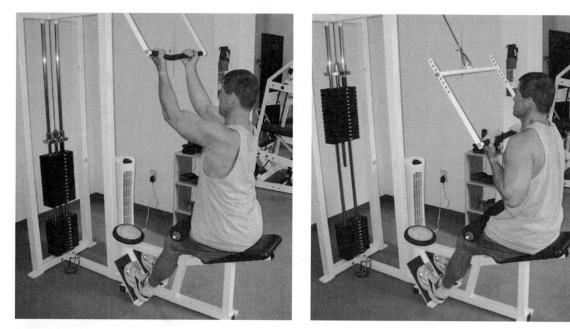

Pulldown (start and finish position)

Pulldown

The next exercise to be performed is the pulldown. Have your arms in front of you, not out to the sides, and use an underhand grip, with your hands a little narrower than shoulder-width apart. This grip is preferred because it provides a slightly greater range of motion than most parallel-grip machines do, in addition to placing the humerus on a plane in front of the body, rather than having it abducted and externally rotated. When the humerus is abducted and externally rotated, it tends to close up the space under the acromion, which is in the shoulder where the glenoid resides, and makes impingement of the structures of the rotator cuff more likely. Having the arms in front of the body also loads the musculature of the frontal torso a bit better, including the abdominal muscles. (See Figure 4.1.)

Muscle Structures Involved. Properly performed, the pulldown exercise thoroughly activates almost all of the musculature of the torso—front and back. Beyond loading the latissimus dorsi muscles of the upper back, this exercise strongly involves other muscle groups. Most notably, the gripping muscles, or forearm flexors, are strongly activated.

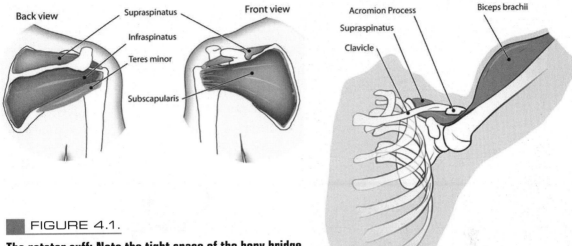

Back view
Front view

Supraspinatus
Infraspinatus
Teres minor
Subscapularis

Acromion Process
Supraspinatus
Clavicle
Biceps brachii

■ FIGURE 4.1.

The rotator cuff: Note the tight space of the bony bridge overhead; any attempt to hold your arm wide during the pulldown (or overhead press) can cause the rotator cuff to be compressed under this bony bridge.

In addition, the biceps is involved to a large degree. Although most train the biceps with single-joint movements such as barbell curls, the biceps crosses both the elbow and shoulder joints, so by doing a pulldown that involves rotation around the elbow and the shoulder joint, you're involving the biceps from both ends. The pulldown further strongly activates the clavicular (upper) portion of the pectoralis muscle, which is involved with initiation of humerus rotation from a stretched position to the contracted position. Note that the first 15 to 20 degrees of motion during the pulldown are initiated by the clavicular portion of the pectoralis.

Pulling hard and keeping your humerus adducted toward the midline heavily involves the pectoralis muscle and even involves the triceps to a large extent. Once your hands are drawn down to a plane even with the top of your head, you are activating the medial head of the triceps to rotate the humerus down toward the plane of the torso. Throughout this range of motion, you're also thoroughly involving the latissimus, the rhomboids, and the trapezius muscles that assist in pulling the bar down. Finally, you will be heavily loading the abdominal muscles, particularly when the slumping motion is employed (as explained in the next section).

Exercise Performance. From a position in which your arms are fully extended above your head, pull the handles (or bar) down to the top of your chest. Hold the contraction for three to five seconds before allowing your arms to return up to the straight position. We typically have our clients keep the torso erect (straight in the seat), and once the handles have been pulled down all the way into the fully contracted position (where the hands are near the top of the chest), we'll instruct them to slump into the contraction. By "slump," we don't mean simply leaning forward, but rather lowering the shoulders directly toward the hips in a linear fashion, as with a vertical crunch. This slumping motion slightly shortens the distance between the sternum and pubic bone by a contraction of the abdominal muscles. When trainees are fully contracted in the slumped position, we have them hold this contraction statically for three to five seconds before relaxing the slump and gradually letting the handles return to the stretched position. As the handles are heading back overhead, we tell trainees to imagine that they're pushing their hands outward in a horizontal plane; this tends to load the latissiumus dorsi muscles more effectively.

Overhead Press

Immediately after the pulldown, you should move on to the overhead press. When this exercise is performed properly, you will be engaging all of the muscles involved in an upper-body "pushing" movement, similar to those involved in the chest press.

Muscle Structures Involved. With the overhead press, you will be strongly involving the triceps muscles, which are on the back of the upper arms, as well as the deltoid musculature and even the pectoralis muscles to a considerable degree. The plane of movement will require the deltoid muscles to be more aggressively recruited earlier in the fatiguing process than the pectoralis muscles; nevertheless, because of orderly recruitment and fatiguing, you're still going to be involving the pectoralis musculature to a significant extent.

Exercise Performance. When performing the overhead press, it is important to move your arms overhead with your hands in front of you, rather than out to the sides, ideally with a parallel grip (palms facing each other).

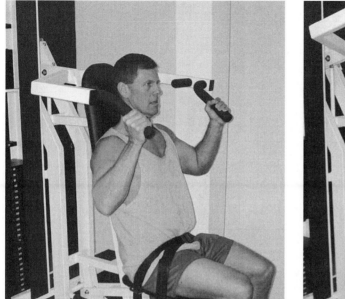 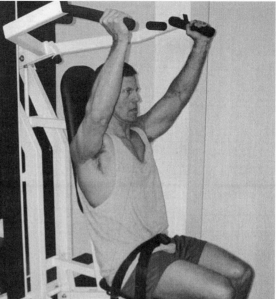

**Overhead press
(start and finish position)**

A parallel grip, particularly when you're performing an upward pushing motion, helps to keep your upper arms adducted toward the midline of your body, as opposed to their being abducted and externally rotated.

If you perform your overhead presses on a machine that requires you to flare your elbows out to your sides (this action is also common in pressing from a behind-the-neck position with a barbell), your arms are abducted outward, and your shoulder is then externally rotated. This is undesirable because it will cause you to rotate the head of the humerus in such a way that its widest part sits underneath the acromion process of the scapula; this produces only a narrow passageway for the rotator cuff tendons to move, as you're pressing your arms up and down, enhancing the risk of impingement syndrome. If you instead perform the overhead press with your arms in a plane in front of your body, with your hands facing each other, you maximize the space between the humeral head and the acromion process, so that the rotator cuff tendons have plenty of room to move without impingement.

As a trainee tires during a set of overhead presses, there is a propensity to arch the lower back to try to acquire more purchase from the shoulder

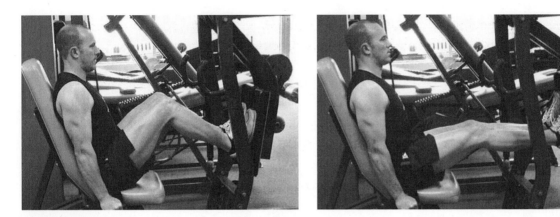

Leg press (start and finish position)

blades against the back pad of the machine. We prefer to have our clients fasten their seat belts for the overhead press and focus instead on pushing the pelvis into the belt, as if they were trying to move their buttocks off the end of the seat. Doing so gives them the purchase they need without requiring them to arch or otherwise place the lower back in a vulnerable position.

Leg Press

The final exercise in the workout is the leg press, which covers virtually every muscle group in the lower body.

Muscle Structures Involved. The leg press exercise hits the entire lower body from the waist down, with particular emphasis on the hip and buttock musculature. It also strongly involves the hamstring musculature on the back of the thighs and the quadriceps musculature located on the front of the thighs, and to some extent, there is also rotation around the ankle joint, which serves to recruit and load the gastrocnemius (calf) muscles of the lower leg. There are many leg press machines from which to choose, with varying pressing angles. Any of them will do the job, but the farther the angle is from linear (straight up and down), the less resistance you are moving (in much the same way that pushing your car horizontally down a street would be much easier than pushing it directly overhead). Exceptions to this would be both Nautilus and MedX leg press machines that make use of offset cams to vary the resistance properly.

Exercise Performance. The leg press machine should be preset so that when you are seated in the machine in the flexed, or tucked, position, your thighs are perpendicular to the ceiling. Your hips should be flexed slightly more than 90 degrees, while your knees should be bent as close to 90 degrees as possible.

Now slowly and smoothly push your legs out to a point just short of lockout. You don't want your knees to be locked out, as this creates a loss of muscle tension during the bone-on-bone tower. From this position, perform a slow transition, or reverse of direction, with your legs now bending until they have returned to the starting position. As you approach the starting position, lightly let the weight touch the weight stack so that it barely makes a "tap," before transitioning back toward the straight-leg position. The movement, inclusive of directional transitions, should be performed in a fluid, smooth, circular motion. Note that it is desirable to take hold of the support handles with a palms-open grip, as the leg press is an exercise in which excessive gripping has no productive purpose and can drive blood pressure levels unnecessarily high.

A Free-Weight Big Five

As not everyone will have access to the machines indicated, the following is a "Big Five" workout that can be performed effectively with free weights.

Bent-Over Barbell Row. Bending over at the waist, take hold of a barbell with a shoulder-width grip. Keep a slight bend in your knees so as not to

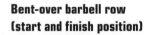

**Bent-over barbell row
(start and finish position)**

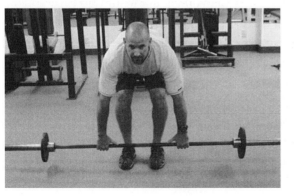
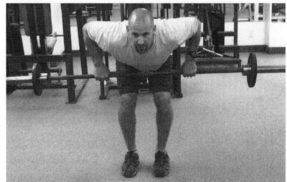

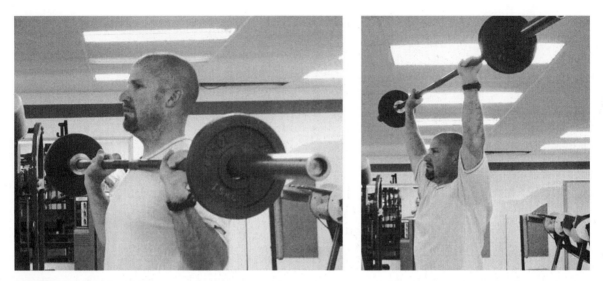

**Standing overhead press
(start and finish position)**

strain your lower back. Slowly draw your arms upward until the bar touches your upper abdomen. Pause briefly in this fully contracted position, and then lower the barbell slowly back to the starting position. Repeat for your time under load. (Note: Time under load, or TUL, is a time signature that should be employed in addition to repetition counting and is explained fully, along with rep speed, following these exercise descriptions.)

Standing Overhead Press. Take hold of a barbell with a shoulder-width grip, and pull it up until you are holding it with your palms facing forward at the front of your shoulders. Keeping your back straight, slowly press the barbell overhead. Unlike with the barbell row, do not pause at the position of full contraction with this exercise, as your arms would be fully locked out, allowing the load to come off the muscles and onto the bone-on-bone tower. Slowly lower the barbell down to your shoulders. Repeat for your TUL.

Dead Lift. Keeping your back straight, bend your legs as if you're sitting down in a chair. Your arms should be kept perfectly straight throughout the performance of this exercise. Take hold of the barbell with a shoulder-width grip. You can grip the barbell either with both hands facing your shins or

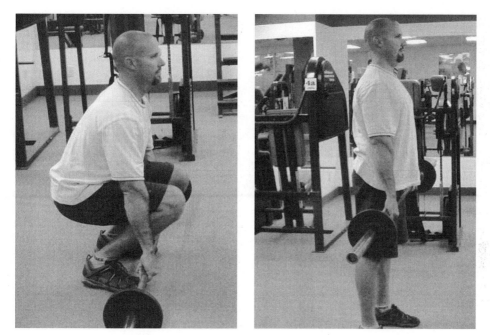

Dead lift (start and finish position)

with an "over/under" grip in which one hand is facing your shins and the other is facing forward. Now, using the strength of your leg muscles, slowly stand up straight so that you are perfectly vertical. Do not rest in this position, but slowly reverse direction, making sure to keep your back straight and your head up, until the bar returns to the starting position. Repeat for your TUL.

Bench Press. To perform this exercise, you will need a flat bench with supports—and, ideally, a power rack. The advantage to using a power rack is that you can set the supports so that when you reach muscular failure, you will not be pinned underneath the barbell. Lying on your back, lift the barbell from the supports and press it up above your chest until your arms are locked out. Do not pause in this position; if you do, as would happen with the overhead press, the load will be transferred onto the bone-on-bone tower that results from locking out your arms, rather than being placed on the musculature responsible for moving your arms into this position. Slowly lower the barbell until it reaches the safety bar of the power rack,

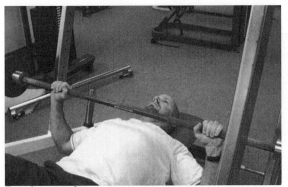
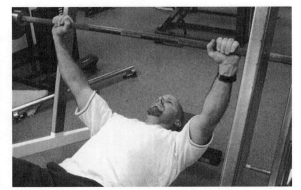

Bench press (start and finish position)

and then slowly press it back to the locked-out position once again. Repeat for your TUL.

Squat. Barbell squats are an excellent lower-body exercise, but the fact that the bar is placed at the nape of one's neck can lead to compression problems. Moreover, hitting a point of muscular failure can be difficult, owing to the fact that unless you are in a power rack or a Smith machine, you could end up pinned and possibly injured.

To perform this exercise, set the safety pins of the power rack at a point that corresponds to a 90-degree bend of your knees. This will represent the bottom position of the movement. Now step under the barbell so that the bar is resting on your trapezius muscle at the base of the neck but not directly on your neck. Straighten your leg so that the barbell is lifted free

Squat (start and finish position)

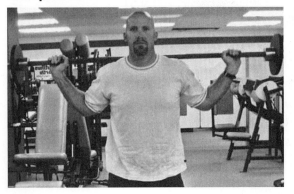
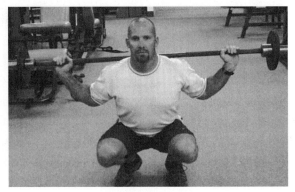

of the support pins (at the top of the rack) that are holding it, and step back. Your feet should be shoulder-width apart, and your back should be straight. Slowly bend your knees, keeping your back straight, until the bar on your shoulders lightly touches the safety pins you have set for 90 degrees. Descend with control, not rapidly. As soon as you lightly touch the safety pins, slowly reverse direction and straighten your legs until you reach the starting position. Repeat for your TUL.

REP SPEED

We advocate that you perform your repetitions in these exercises slowly. Data accumulated from the scientific literature overwhelmingly indicate that moving faster diminishes strength gains.[2] The reason is that with faster performance, momentum has contributed to the movement of the weight, as opposed to muscle fiber involvement.[3] In a study conducted by physiologist Wayne Wescott, a director of strength training for the YMCA, male and female subjects between twenty-five and eighty-two years of age were put into two groups, one that trained in a slow fashion and one that trained in a faster, more conventional manner. Over a ten-week period, the subjects in the slower-contraction group showed a 59 percent increase in overall strength, compared with a 39 percent increase for the faster-contraction group.[4]

Your goal is not simply moving a weight from point A to point B, but rather the inroading, or weakening, of muscle. The more effectively you can load a muscle, the more efficiently you will inroad it. In addition to building more strength, training with a more controlled cadence significantly reduces the risk of injury.[5] Therefore, in terms of both efficaciousness and delivering a better stimulus for positive adaptation, slower is better.

How slowly should you lift and lower weights? We advise that you move the weight as slowly as you possibly can without the movement degenerating into a series of starts and stops. How slow that cadence will be depends on the accuracy of the strength curves of the equipment you're using, how much friction is in the equipment, and your natural neurological efficiency. Some trainees will find that they can move perfectly smoothly with a cadence of fifteen seconds up, fifteen seconds down, which is fine. Others will find that they can't use any rep cadence slower than five seconds up and five seconds down without their repetitions becoming herky-jerky affairs.

Our rule of thumb for rep cadence is that whatever cadence you can employ that will allow you to move as slowly as possible without its turning into a stuttering, stop-and-start scenario is the right one for you. You may even find that the cadence changes as the set progresses. For instance, if you're working out on a piece of equipment that has a difficult start but an easy finish position, the hard start will represent a significant obstacle or sticking point to surmount. Consequently, you may start out with an eight-second cadence that is perfectly smooth, but because of the sticking point and a little bit of struggle, the smoothness may be able to be maintained only with a six-second cadence or a five-second cadence. So, again, contract against the resistance as slowly as you can without having your repetitions degenerate into a series of stops and starts.

Time Under Load (TUL)

Traditionally during workouts, to gauge performance and assess improvement for record keeping, trainees have focused on counting how many repetitions they perform with a given weight or load. What we advocate instead is timing the duration of the set from the moment it begins until the moment muscular failure is reached. We call this measure "time under load." Other people have called it "time to concentric failure" or "time under tension." Regardless of what you choose to call it, adopting it allows you to place a fine-tuning dial on your training performance.

If, for instance, you end up averaging ten seconds up and ten seconds down, that would be twenty seconds during which your muscles are under load within the context of a given repetition. Now, if you reached failure at six reps in an exercise during one workout and six reps the next, but your time under load was a minute and thirty seconds during the first workout and a minute and forty seconds during the next workout, you would have missed that ten-second display of increased strength by merely counting repetitions. Time under load allows trainees to see smaller gradations in improvement that otherwise might be missed and allows for fine-tuning of weight progression a little more closely.

BREATHING

Breathing throughout the performance of each exercise should be continuous and natural, and it should be performed with an open mouth. As an exercise becomes more difficult and the lactic acid begins to accumulate in your muscles, causing that "burning" sensation, you should deliberately breathe faster, or hyperventilate. This step will help you break the urge to hold your breath and employ the Valsalva maneuver (the holding of one's breath while exerting; technically it's a closing of the glottis or vocal chords, or getting a gulp of air in the chest and then pushing hard against it). We don't want to you to do this, for several reasons:

1. It unnecessarily raises blood pressure.
2. It raises intravascular pressure on the venous circulation.
3. It increases intrathoracic pressure, which decreases venous return to the heart.
4. Within muscle, it provides an internal mechanical assist, which is why power lifters will hold their breath in straining to make record lifts. However, doing so undermines our goal of fatiguing and inroading the muscle, as it essentially short-circuits that process. So, not only is it a potentially dangerous thing to do, it also runs counter to the inroading process that we're trying to achieve.

RIDING OUT THE STORM (UNDERSTANDING THE INROAD PROCESS)

The stimulus for positive adaptive change has many factors. Clearly, there is a strong cardiovascular component, as your cardiorespiratory system services the mechanical functioning of your muscles. Thus, the higher the intensity of muscular work, the higher the degree of cardiovascular and respiratory stimulation. There is also a large production of accumulated by-products of fatigue, in that metabolic wastes such as lactic acid accumulate faster than they can be eliminated by the body. These effects create an environment in which certain growth factors are released and

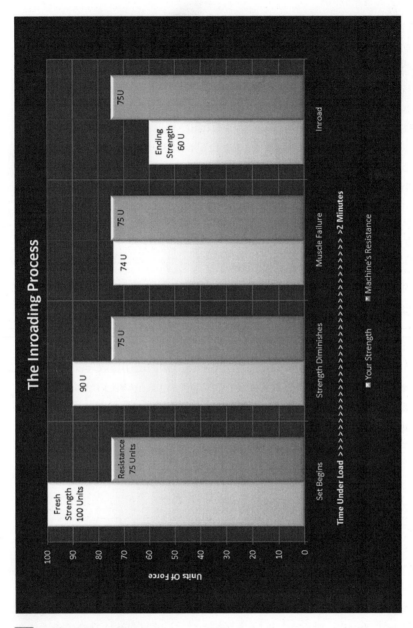

FIGURE 4.2.

This graph illustrates what happens to your strength as you perform a set of exercises. Time is along the bottom (x-axis), and units of force are along the side (y-axis). The gray bars represent the machine's resistance (weights) steady at 75 units. Each set of white bars indicates the progression of the set and the ever-weakening strength of your muscles.

the first stages of muscle growth are stimulated.[6] Load, or weight, is a part of this process as well. Exposure to heavier weights causes microscopic cellular damage that initiates the muscular adaptation and seems to be essential for stimulating increases in both muscle and bone mineral density.[7]

All of these factors are present and contribute to the stimulation process when the mechanism of inroading, or weakening, of the muscles is employed. High-intensity muscular contractions, during the course of which muscle tissue is made to weaken, is a powerful stimulus for positive change.[8] It is crucial, therefore, for all trainees to have a firm intellectual understanding of what it is that they are striving to achieve. We have found it helpful to use the inroading diagram (Figure 4.2) to help explain this process.

At the beginning of a set, your strength is untapped; let's call it 100 units of force. You will not choose 100 units of resistance, however, but rather 75 units, to oppose your strength. For inroading to occur, the resistance to which you expose your muscles must be meaningful, which is between 75 percent and 80 percent of your starting level of strength. If the resistance you select is too light, your muscles will recover at a faster rate than they fatigue, with the result that no inroading will occur. Using a slow protocol, you will proceed to perform your repetitions, moving the weights up and down. (We would typically have you employ ten seconds on the positive, or lifting, phase and ten seconds on the negative, or lowering, assuming that the equipment has correct cam profiles and low friction.) This slower speed of lifting eliminates momentum, increases safety, and keeps your muscles under load for the duration of the set.

With each passing moment, your strength diminishes, with the result that your force output is now starting to drop, and your rate of fatigue and fiber involvement increases. You have now lost some of your initial 100 units of strength, but your muscles are still stronger than the 75 units of resistance that you are lifting and lowering. You are now perceiving that the repetitions are getting harder. Your body instinctively doesn't like to be fatigued so quickly, and you are starting to receive negative feedback, which typically manifests in a fervent desire to quit the exercise. Nevertheless, you soldier on, attempting to maintain a continual loading of your muscles and increase your concentration so as not to break form and unload your muscles. As the difficulty level increases, you may grow anxious as you sense that muscular failure is approaching. (This anxiety is a normal reaction.)

You will begin to really struggle at this point, and your instructor should try to keep you focused by encouraging you not to try to speed up, rest, or pause during the movement, all of which will unload the muscles and provide rest, which is the opposite of what you are striving to accomplish. If you weren't being supervised, you would probably quit at this juncture, but you are encouraged to try one more repetition. This last positive portion of the repetition is now so difficult that it may take you fifteen, twenty, or even thirty seconds to complete. As you slowly begin to reverse direction and lower the resistance, the weight begins to overtake your strength. You attempt another positive repetition, but the weight is not moving. Your instructor now tells you to attempt to contract against the resistance (it's still not moving) while he or she counts to ten. Your rate of fatigue is increasing rapidly now, and your strength continues to diminish well below the resistance level. At the end of the instructor's count, you unload from the weight. By the time the set is finished, your strength has been reduced to approximately 60 percent of what it was prior to starting the exercise, resulting in an inroad of 40 percent being made.

This whole process occurred over a span of roughly two minutes, but in that time, your muscles became 40 percent weaker. This occurrence represents a serious "threat" to your body, because it was not aware that you were simply in a gym making weights go up and down. For all it knew, you were fighting for your life with a mountain lion. To the body, this was a profound metabolic experience, and at the end of that experience, *it couldn't move*. Mobility is a preserved biologic function: if you can't move, you can't acquire food, and you can't avoid becoming food for other prey. This experience represented a profound stimulus, to which the body will respond, if given sufficient time, by enlarging on its strength reserves so that there will be at least some strength left over the next time such a stimulus might be encountered. Of course, now that you understand this process, you will employ slightly more resistance during your next workout to stimulate your body to produce another round of metabolic adaptation.

Bear in mind that as you fatigue during this process, and as your force output drops, you will feel the window between your force output and the resistance you're using starting to close. You'll develop an almost instinctual sense of panic, a feeling that you're not strong enough to meet the resistance you're under. This is the "make-or-break" point in the set. If you understand that what you're trying to do is achieve a deep level of muscular fatigue, you can override the instinct to attempt to escape. Escape in this context can take the form either of prematurely quitting and just shutting down or of attempting to wiggle and jab at the weight to momentarily get out from under the load.

We tell our clients, "We don't care if the weight bogs down, and we don't care if it stops moving. Just keep pushing in the same manner that you did in the beginning, and if it stops moving, don't panic: just keep pushing. It's not important at the end if the repetition is completed." An understanding that your instincts run counter to achieving this degree of fatigue, and that you have to intellectually override your instincts in order to achieve it, is crucial. The most important thing for you to grasp is the nature of the process. To be able to push to the point where physical activity becomes a stimulus for productive change, it helps to understand that it's OK to feel a little anxious or panicky during the set. After all, the purpose of the exercise is not to make the weight go up and down; it is to achieve a deep level of inroad, to reach the point where you can no longer move the weight but still keep trying. If you have that degree of intellectual understanding, then you will be able to override the instincts that otherwise would intercede to prevent you from stimulating the production of a positive adaptive response from your body.

Muscular Failure

A logical question arises: What point of fatigue should the beginner target? Is it the point at which another repetition isn't possible? Or is it—at least during the first few workouts—simply the point of discomfort? It has been our experience that most clients, even beginners, should try to go to a point of positive failure right from the get-go. If you find that you have misjudged the resistance you should be using and are performing the exercise for too long (more than ninety seconds), keep going until you hit positive failure, and increase the weight by approximately 5 to 10 percent (or whatever amount is required) to get you back under the ninety-second time under load.

Admittedly, there will be trainees who are or have been sedentary and therefore are not used to exerting themselves. For them, the entire concept of inroading their muscles will represent such foreign territory that sometimes they'll quit the exercise well before they've reached a point of positive failure. In such instances, we use their point of voluntary shutdown as a tentative definition of positive "failure" for a workout or two, until they start to develop a skill set and better tolerance for exertional discomfort that allows them to go to true muscular failure. Otherwise, if clients are able, we will have them go to failure right from the outset.

A lot of times, that failure point will be determined by the trainee's current capabilities and level of toleration of exertional discomfort. Once an individual gets acclimated to this condition, we encourage inroading to the point of momentary muscular failure (positive failure). We believe that this is safe to do, because what you can bring to yourself is pretty much limited by your current capabilities; you can never bring more to yourself than you're capable of handling.

Frequency

A trainee who is relatively well conditioned and is going to true failure should perform the Big-Five workout once every seven days. There are exceptions: the recovery interval needs to be predicated on the individual's level of intensity during the initial workout and the muscle-mass level at baseline. A petite, 100-pound woman whose intensity level is such that her failure level is determined by her toleration of discomfort could easily work out twice a week and not have any concerns about overtraining. Then again, a relatively athletic young male who weighs a solid 170 pounds and is able to go to true muscular failure may need to work out only once every seven to ten days. Even that 100-pound woman will eventually have to add recovery days to her time off between workouts as she grows stronger, until she too is training only once a week or less frequently.

The seven-day rest is predicated on the absolute mechanical work that a person is performing: are the weights significant, and is the metabolic cost high? A person who is not capable initially of performing enough mechanical/metabolic work to make that seven-day recovery a requisite may initially benefit from slightly more frequent training, but otherwise, all things being equal, once every seven days is an excellent frequency with which to start.

If you're doing everything appropriately—working hard enough, keeping the volume of the workout in the realm in which your recovery can manage it, and keeping proper track of your performance—the amount of resistance you're using should progress in a stepwise fashion, and you should be matching or bettering your time under load at an increasing resistance from workout to workout. Once that situation stops occurring, and you are starting to have difficulty with progression, that is an early marker that you need to start inserting more recovery days, because you are now accumulating enough strength to produce enough of a workload that it is proving difficult for you to recover at that particular frequency.

It has been our observation that, by and large, people who come to a personal training facility want to get going with a program and settle into a routine. Often enough, if you just settle them into the routine, and they get used to "This is my appointment time on this day, and this is when I exercise," long-term compliance is established right from square one. Most commercial health clubs turn over the vast majority of the people they sign up in less than twelve weeks, whereas the average person in our facilities has been there for four to seven years, and some of them have been there for ten years, because the compliance is enhanced by a manageable volume, frequency, and regularity that becomes a comfortable component of their lifestyle.

Rest Periods Between Exercises

We encourage our clients to move quickly from one exercise to the next. Thirty seconds to a minute is typical for them to make the move and get adjusted into the next piece of equipment. There are metabolic conditioning benefits to be achieved by moving briskly. As you accumulate the by-products of fatigue, the amount of resistance that you can use drops, so the relative degree of inroad that you're achieving as you progress through the workout is increased.

Ideally, you should move briskly enough from exercise to exercise that you're huffing and puffing and not inclined to carry on a conversation with your instructor or workout partner. The pace should be such that you produce a fairly profound metabolic effect, but you shouldn't move so quickly that you feel light-headed or nauseated. At the other extreme, you shouldn't pace yourself to the point where you feel so completely recovered that it's as if you're starting the first set of a workout sequence on every movement.

Record Keeping

The workout record sheet should be standardized. There should be a space for the date of the workout, the time of the workout, what exercises are performed, how much resistance was used, seat position (where applicable), and cadence employed—or time under load. It's also not a bad idea to record the elapsed time from when the first exercise commenced until failure was reached on the last exercise in the program.

If you are keeping track of your time under load, you may also find it helpful to keep a record of the difference between the total accumulated TULs and the elapsed time of the workout, in order to keep rest intervals fairly constant. This is done by noting the elapsed time of the workout and then totaling all the TULs for the workout and subtracting that number from the elapsed time. The remainder will equal your total rest time for all of the movements for that workout. That figure should also not display massive increases. For example, if your workout record reveals big improvements in performance, but when you look at your total time under load minus the elapsed time, you find that your total rest time for the workout has increased by five minutes, then maybe your performance hasn't increased by as much as you thought it had.

WHEN IS THE PROGRAM CHANGED?

It is advisable to stay on this program, as is, for anywhere from four to twelve weeks, depending on how you are progressing. Should you notice a slowdown in your progress, then we would advise breaking the program down into just one upper-body pulling exercise, one upper-body pushing exercise, and a leg press. Alternatively, you could choose one of the Big-Three movements (pulldown, chest press, or leg press; or bent-over barbell row, bench press, or squat, if you're using free weights) and two peripherals. These can be smaller, rotary-type movements that have less of an impact on recovery. In other words, you could select a movement from the Big Three plus two smaller isolation exercises. Likewise, if you aren't filled with any mental angst about doing only three exercises, then just cutting the five-exercise workout to a three-exercise workout, consisting of a pushing movement, a pulling movement, and a leg press, would be fine.

This workout will effectively stimulate all of the major muscular structures within the body. It does not comprise dozens of exercises that will chew up time on a clock. It focuses on the best exercises for all-around bodily strength and function. For time-efficient, productive exercise, this is the most effective program we have found. It has stimulated the most dramatic and significant results in the health and fitness of our clients.

The Benefits of the Big-Five Workout

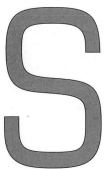

o, now that you have an effective exercise program, what exactly are you accomplishing by employing it? The simple answer is that if your resistance training is properly executed, and the result is the building of muscle, the ultimate gain to the human body is literally "everything."

The metabolic subsystems that support an increased musculature increase their functional capacity along with the size of the muscles that employ them. The closer you get to realizing your muscular potential, the closer you get to optimizing the potential of your metabolic system or "support system." The "health" territory that muscle tissue covers is phenomenal. It includes the potential for processing waste materials, oxygenating blood, controlling insulin levels, optimizing bone-mineral density, increasing metabolic rate, reducing bodyfat levels, optimizing aerobic capacity, enhancing flexibility, and appreciably reducing the chances of injury, while at the same time allowing you to perform day-to-day tasks with far less wear and tear and stress on your body. All of these health benefits flow from the building and strengthening of your muscles.

Vee Ferguson, who is forty-three years old, is a high-intensity-training client of trainer Bo Railey. Over the course of three years of training with four or five exercises once every seven days, he has lost more than 70 pounds of bodyfat and gotten into the best shape of his life.

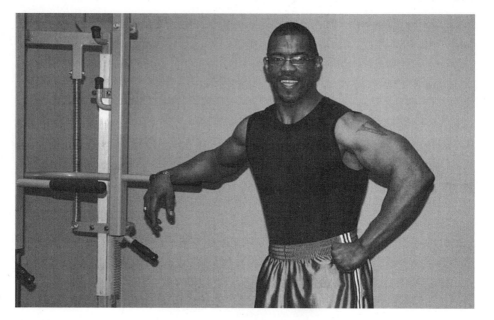

An increase in muscle mass allows you to move from where you are right now in regard to health to what is in your genetic potential for you to become. The closer you move toward the fulfillment of your genetic potential, the more "health" benefits you will enjoy. However, health can be only below, at, or slightly above the baseline, relative to what your muscular potential is at present. There is no "superhealth," and there is no chance that you will experience either the fitness or the health of someone whose genetics for such qualities you don't share, and vice versa. Nevertheless, to someone who is residing below baseline in muscular fitness and potential, the fulfillment of muscular potential—which could be several points above a "normal" baseline level of health—can be the difference between a dreary life of frustration, pain, and chronic anxiety and a life of enjoyment, options, less stress, and no pain. Properly performed exercise is the vehicle that will move you closer to the fulfillment of this potential.

When we say that proper exercise can enhance flexibility, cardiovascular functioning, and strength, we're really saying that it can fulfill your potential in these areas of human functional ability and can thus optimize the functioning of the various support systems of human muscle. That's what this book is about. With that goal in mind, the following sections describe in what way proper exercise will enhance or optimize these various components of a healthy and fit human body.

MORE MUSCLE CAN SAVE YOUR LIFE

The medical literature affirms the absolute role that increased muscle mass plays to one's benefit during life-threatening situations. A lot of the beneficial effects of strength training come from the fact that other organs of the body increase their functional capacity to track, one to one, with increases in muscle mass. As an example, if you were to be in a severe traffic accident and had to be admitted to an intensive care unit, the "start" point from which you would atrophy all of your organs is predicated on your degree of muscle mass. In other words, how long it would take before you reach multisystem organ failure and die is directly linked to your level of muscle mass, because all of your other organ weights are going to be proportional to that.

Saving Lives with High-Intensity Training

A physician colleague of mine had severe emphysema. One night, he was brought into the emergency room of the hospital where I was on duty. Though he was in respiratory failure, he didn't want to be put on a ventilator. As a colleague and a friend, I sat down with him and said, "Look, if we don't put you on a ventilator, then you are going to die—and you're going to die *tonight*. I know you don't want to be on a ventilator. I know you're worried about suffering, being on life support for weeks on end, and then eventually dying anyway, but if you can get through this one OK, I think that you can have many more years of productive life ahead of you."

He reluctantly agreed, and for a time, I felt bad for talking him into it, because he did spend two weeks on a ventilator, and when he eventually got off, he was for the most part wheelchair bound because of his emphysema. He could walk short distances inside his house, and on a good day, he could walk out to his mailbox or onto his driveway to pick up the newspaper, but he was in bad shape and getting worse.

Then, out of the blue, he decided to come to my training facility. He said that he wanted to work out, so I put him on the Big Three routine consisting of a pulldown, chest press, and leg press. This routine gradually strengthened him. With his increasing muscle strength, the amount of respiratory support he required to accomplish a given level of muscular exertion started to fall—because he was stronger. He worked out once a week, and we trained him to the point where we doubled his strength. As a result, when he needed his muscles to perform a level of work that previously would have required him to recruit all of his available motor units and left him exhausted, he now had to recruit only half that amount. Consequently, his heart and lungs now had to support the work of only half the motor units that they had to before, which amounted to far less work for his respiratory system.

Rather than dying that night in the ER, my colleague lived for another six years, and he lived a fully functional and ambulatory life, never requiring a wheelchair again. He ended up taking not one, but two, world cruises with his wife, and he didn't have to take along a wheelchair. He was able to see all the sights and experience all the adventures that everybody else did, despite almost having died several months earlier, simply because he was stronger.

Muscle is the body's richest source of mitochondria, the oxygen-producing component of all cellular tissue. It's definitely where you have the most opportunity for metabolic adaptation, and more of it is produced by your increasing the amount of muscle on your body through the performance of proper strength training.

—Doug McGuff, M.D.

STRENGTH

Exercise that is performed to make your muscles bigger also makes them stronger (and vice versa). When you're stronger, the metabolic consequence of any work that you have to do as part of your daily life becomes less significant. Having more strength benefits you in all activities; it not only makes everything you do easier but also broadens the scope of what you can do.

The first thing that most of our clients notice, even before they see changes in the mirror, is that they are now able to perform some feat that they were previously not able to do. For instance, a middle-aged woman will remark, "I was at the grocery store, and I picked up a fifty-pound bag of dog food with one hand and moved it from the shopping cart to the trunk of my car. And then it hit me: Holy cow! Did I just do that?" Similarly, other people will report day-to-day gains in going about their regular activities such as gardening, cleaning, performing home repairs, and just climbing steps. One gentleman who trains with us lives on a nice lake and enjoys boating, but he has a long walk down two flights of steps to his dock. To keep his boat fueled, he has to carry two heavy gas tanks down these stairs and customarily had to stop after the first flight to rest. Shortly after he started strength training, he was able to make it all the way down to his boat without stopping once and without feeling winded or exerted.

GASTROINTESTINAL TRANSIT TIME

Slow gastrointestinal transit time has been associated with a higher risk of colon cancer, and gastrointestinal transit time has been shown to increase by as much as 56 percent after just three months of strength-training exercise.[1] So, again, the greater your muscle mass, the quicker the gastrointestinal transit time and, therefore, the lower your risk for colon cancer.

Resting metabolism

Muscle is metabolically active tissue. Any loss of muscle with age leads to a lower energy requirement and a reduced resting metabolic rate. Without proper strength-training exercise to intercede, the resting metabolic rate will diminish by approximately 2 to 5 percent per decade.[2] A study conducted by Tufts University in which senior men and women took part in a twelve-week basic strength-building program resulted in the subjects' gaining an average of three pounds of lean muscle weight and reducing their bodyfat weight by an average of four pounds. As a consequence, the resting metabolic rate of the subjects increased by 7 percent, on average, which was the equivalent of an additional 108 calories burned per day, or an extra 756 calories per week. This study indicated that the body burns at least 35 calories a day for every pound of lean muscle weight gained. This new tissue will burn more calories even while the subject is at rest. (Fat, by contrast requires about 2 calories a day per pound for the body to sustain.)[3]

Glucose metabolism

The ability to metabolize glucose efficiently is vital to health. Diabetes has been associated with poor glucose metabolism, which strength training has been shown to improve, increasing glucose uptake by 23 percent after only four months.[4]

Insulin sensitivity

Human beings require periodic bursts of high muscular effort. In the absence of such activity, glycogen is not drained out of the muscles to any meaningful degree. When this state is coupled with routine consumption of large amounts of refined carbohydrates, a level of glucose is produced that can no longer be stored in the muscles. The muscles are already full, because an insufficient number of glycolytic fibers have been tapped. Glucose therefore begins to stack up in the bloodstream, and the body's insulin levels rise. Because the glucose cannot get into the muscle cells, the receptors on the surface of those cells become insensitive to insulin. The body then produces even *more* insulin and now has large amounts of circulating glucose *and* large amounts of circulating insulin. That glucose gets transported to the liver, where, in the face of high insulin levels, it will attach to fatty acids (triacylglycerol), and all future carbohydrate ingestion now is partitioned exclusively to fat storage.

Long after your muscle cells have become insensitive to insulin, your fat cells (adipocytes) remain sensitive to insulin. As a result, the system of someone who does not perform high-energy exercise will have high amounts of triacylglycerol, which is then moved into the fat cells, where it is converted to triglycerides and ends up being stored as bodyfat.

One of the most important ways to reverse this process is to engage in physical activity that is intense enough that it taps into the higher-order fibers where glycogen storage is greatest. This occurrence causes the release of adrenaline, or epinephrine, which creates an amplification cascade that cleaves large amounts of glycogen out of the cell. The reason glycogen is stored in the muscle is for emergency utilization, on site, for fight-or-flight situations. High-intensity training accomplishes this in a way that no other form of physical activity can even approximate, triggering a release of adrenaline that cleaves tens of thousands of molecules of gylcogen for immediate on-site burning by the musculature. This process creates room for glycogen to enter the muscle cell.

Now the glucose that was previously stacking up in the bloodstream can be moved into the muscle cell, and the insulin receptors on the muscles can operate and start to become more sensitive. As they become more insulin sensitive, the glucose levels in the bloodstream diminish, and the insulin levels in the bloodstream fall concurrently.

RELEASE OF BODYFAT STORES

Bodyfat loss is another benefit that proper strength training affords the trainee. This benefit of a resistance-training program is a result of three factors. The first is that an increase in muscle mass raises the resting metabolic rate of the body, thus burning more calories in a twenty-four-hour period. The second is that calories are burned during the strength-training activity as well as being burned, and at a higher rate, following the cessation of the workout while the body undergoes replenishment of exhausted energy reserves and repairs damaged tissues. Third, as discussed, while the muscles empty themselves of glycogen, glucose is moved out of the bloodstream and into the muscle, lowering the bloodstream's insulin levels. When this happens, the amount of triacylglycerol in the liver and in the circulation falls. This lower insulin level translates to *less* bodyfat storage.

This third component is a process that occurs in both directions almost completely irrespective of calorie balance. That's why when morbidly obese people are put on low-calorie diets but are not performing high-intensity exercise, and their carbohydrates are not restricted enough to affect their insulin levels, they find it *impossible* to lose bodyfat.

The substance responsible for mobilizing bodyfat is hormone-sensitive lipase, which is especially sensitive to both epinephrine and insulin. In the face of epinephrine, hormone-sensitive lipase will mobilize fatty acids out of the fat cells for emergency energy usage, but in the presence of insulin, the action of hormone-sensitive lipase is inhibited. When you perform high-intensity strength training, epinephrine stimulates an amplification cascade of hormone-sensitive lipase, allowing the liberation of fatty acids from the fat cells, to begin the fat-mobilization process. This outcome is a dividend of high-intensity exercise itself, irrespective of calorie balance.

CHOLESTEROL (BLOOD LIPID) LEVELS

High-intensity strength training has been shown to have a positive effect on cholesterol levels, improving blood lipid profiles after only a few weeks of strength-training exercise.[5] To a large extent, insulin plays a role here as well, as it is a pro-inflammatory hormone, which, in combination with high levels of glucose, results in more oxidative damage to tissue. A generalized inflammatory state is created, marked by a lot of inflammation on the walls of the blood vessels, which now must be repaired. Cholesterol is a ubiquitous hormone within the body, the equivalent of biologic mortar or spackle; when an inflammatory condition develops on the blood vessel wall, that inflammation is patched over with cholesterol.

Low-density lipoprotein (LDL) and *high-density lipoprotein* (HDL) basically refer to the density of the protein that is carrying the cholesterol. To understand how these two lipoproteins operate, one has to examine how blood flows. The flow rate in the central portion of a vessel is slightly higher than the flow rate at its periphery. Just as leaves in a river tend to flow out to the edges of the banks, metabolites of lower density tend to behave that way in the bloodstream. Consequently, when the body needs to take cholesterol out to the blood vessel walls to mortar up an inflamed area, it is going to deploy LDL cholesterol to patch the inflammatory sites.

If, on the other hand, the body needs to bring cholesterol back to the liver for processing, this is best accomplished through the central circulation, where it's not going to stick to the cell walls. HDL cholesterol, therefore, is deployed in such situations, bringing any circulating insulin to the central circulation for processing into other elements, including the synthesis of hormones. In this instance, your body requires a high-density lipoprotein to carry the cholesterol through the central portion of the blood vessel, rather than its periphery. So, the ratio of HDL to LDL is largely an indirect marker of the body's generalized inflammatory state. Restoring insulin sensitivity decreases that systemic inflammatory state, which results in a less-generalized inflammation of blood vessel walls, thus requiring less need for cholesterol to be transported for this purpose on LDL molecules.

Viewed in this light, high cholesterol levels are really a symptom, not a cause of cardiovascular disease. Not understanding this fact, a lot of people take medicine to try to lower their LDL cholesterol levels artificially. Attempting to control through medication the enzymes that produce elevated cholesterol is analogous to playing pool with a rope. The practical course is to treat the cause of the elevated cholesterol levels by correcting the underlying cellular inflammation, so that the stimulus to produce the LDL is weaker and the stimulus to produce the HDL is stronger. Those levels are basically indirect markers, or downstream effects, of your generalized inflammatory state, which is largely related to the amount of circulating glucose and insulin in the body.

Diet also plays a role here, of course. Eating a proper diet is a giant first step in correcting the whole metabolic syndrome. Consuming a hunter-gatherer type of diet that is relatively restricted in carbohydrates and exceedingly restricted in refined carbohydrates, which cause high spikes in glucose and insulin, can have a profound effect on all of these parameters. The effect derives from your favoring glucagon over insulin, but diet alone is not sufficient, because glucagon works on a nonamplifying mechanism, whereby one molecule of glucagon will affect one molecule of glucose.

The true remedy is, once again, high-intensity exercise. Only it has a significant effect on insulin sensitivity, due to the amplification cascade it produces, which aggressively empties glycogen out of the muscles, creating a situation in which enhanced insulin sensitivity becomes a necessity. You have to work out at a level high enough to prompt the glycolytic cells to empty their stores of glycogen. You're not going to accomplish this by diet alone, by walking on a treadmill, or by a steady-state jog. That's because for any given level of glucose ingested, the amount of insulin that has to be secreted to resolve the situation is much, much lower.

BLOOD PRESSURE

Increased blood pressure is a growing health concern for many middle-aged people. It had long been supposed that the effort involved with weight training could be problematic for people suffering from high blood pressure. However, the medical literature reveals that properly performed strength training has actually been shown to *reduce* resting blood pressure in mildly hypertensive adults without the risk of dangerous blood pressure increase.[6]

BONE MINERAL DENSITY

There is no shortage of data in the medical literature indicating that significant increases in bone mineral density can be derived from strength training.[7] Not only will proper strength training make you stronger, but also this strength helps to protect you from sustaining the sorts of falls that cause the types of fractures we witness in osteoporosis sufferers. Moreover, should you experience such a fall, if you're stronger and your muscle mass is significant, the additional muscle will function as a force-dissipating agent to protect your bones. It is in areas such as this that proper strength training asserts itself as a superior means of exercise, especially with senior citizens. Jogging, walking, playing golf, running on treadmills, and the like do not provide enough of a meaningful load to cause the body to grow more protective muscle. Even lightweight exercises are ineffective in this regard. In one study, fifty-six subjects were randomized to either heavy or light resistance training; only the group that performed their resistance training with heavier loads increased their bone mineral density.[8]

While strength training can be a helpful activity to combat osteoporosis, there is some reason to believe that the loss of bone mineral density with age is an entirely hormonally mediated trait and thus may not be affected by exercise. If this is true, it nevertheless follows that if you appropriately strengthen your muscles, the actual bone mineral density of these critical areas will become almost moot. If the surrounding supporting musculature is strong enough, you can tolerate large losses in bone density with lesser consequences. Evidence comes from a joint study conducted by Yale University Medical School and Hokkaido Medical School (Japan), in which the author of the study, Manohar Pahjabi, concluded:

> The human spinal column devoid of musculature is incapable of carrying the physiological loads imposed on it. It has been shown experimentally that an isolated fresh cadaveric spinal column from T 1 to the sacrum placed in an upright neutral position with sacrum fixed to the test table can carry a load of not more than 20 N before it buckles and becomes unstable. Therefore, muscles are necessary to stabilize the spine so that it can carry out its normal physiologic functions.[9]

Arthur Jones, who spent years studying the mechanics and musculature of the lower back, confirmed this finding, claiming that a twenty-year-old human spine devoid of its supporting musculature would collapse under the weight equivalent of a can of soda. So, many hip breaks are probably attributable to the fact that the surrounding supporting musculature was too weak to serve its shock-absorber function and thus unable to effectively dissipate the force that caused the breakage.

SYMPTOMS OF ARTHRITIS

People who suffer from arthritis will be pleased to learn that strength-training research on arthritic subjects has shown that resistance exercise may ease the discomfort of both osteoarthritis and rheumatoid arthritis.[10] In one study, the researchers concluded: "High intensity strength training is feasible and safe in selected patients with well-controlled rheumatoid arthritis and leads to significant improvements in strength, pain, and fatigue without exacerbating disease activity or joint pain."[11]

LOWER-BACK PAIN

One of the more common ailments we witness in contemporary society is lower-back pain. Fortunately, there is strong medical evidence that a properly performed resistance-training program involving direct exercise for the muscles of the lumbar spine can help to ease lower-back discomfort and to strengthen the lumbar muscles. In a study involving patients with either radicular or referred leg pain, more than half of all subjects responded to strength training just as well as patients with isolated low-back pain. What made this study interesting for our purposes was the fact that prior to evaluation at a Physicians Neck and Back Clinic (PNBC), these patients had seen on average three physicians and had failed six different treatment options, comprising chiropractic, epidural injections, facet injections, ultrasound, traction, medication, and electrical stimulation. The patients who completed the PNBC had 67 percent less medical reutilization in the year after discharge than comparable control-group patients treated elsewhere with passive modalities.[12]

In a combined study between the PNBC and the University of California, San Diego, that used resistance training only, the experimenters were able to achieve comparable excellent results with comparable spine patients. Moreover, health care reutilization was dramatically reduced at both clinics to almost identical levels, which further validated the results of each. In the year after completing the strength-training treatment, only 12 percent of the PNBC patients needed to reenter the health care system as a result of their spinal problems.[13] In addition, a study of patients suffering lower-back problems who performed twelve weeks of specific strength-training exercise for the lower-back muscles found that the subjects experienced significantly less lower-back discomfort.[14]

FLEXIBILITY

In most instances, people consider flexibility to be the third leg of the fitness tripod, the other two being cardiovascular stimulation and strength building. While enhanced flexibility is desirable, you don't have to enroll in a yoga class or stretch constantly (or at all) to safely achieve flexibility. There is widespread confusion, even among fitness authorities, between stretching and flexibility. What you want is not *increased* flexibility so much as *enhanced* flexibility. This goal is achieved by an application of resistance at the safe extremes of a muscle's range of motion.

In a study conducted on young people who performed a strength-training program, the experimenters concluded that the strength-trained subjects were able to improve their range of movement far more than were the control subjects.[15] In another study, forty-eight subjects who performed Nautilus strength training over a period of eight weeks improved their hip-trunk flexibility by two and a half inches without performing any stretching exercises, while simultaneously increasing muscle strength by 50 percent.[16]

In setting up an appropriate resistance-training program, the selected exercises should track muscle and joint function and apply resistance through full flexion to full extension. Built into proper resistance exercise is an application of force at the extremes of a muscle's (or muscle group's) safe range of motion. For some joints, this may mean that we're going to improve or increase the range of that joint, but for other joints, an enhanced flexibility may actually result in a decrease in that joint's range of motion. Most of the problems and derangements that occur in the shoulder joint, for example, are a result not of inadequate flexibility but of *excessive* flexibility. The increased strength and development of the surrounding rotator cuff muscles, as well as the deltoid musculature, may diminish the range of the shoulder joint somewhat, but in a way that is protective to the joint.

It follows that by performing appropriate exercise with resistance through a full range of motion, you will be doing everything that you should (and could) to improve your flexibility. Yoga or stretching exercises are not going to enhance your flexibility. Instead, either they will induce a state of sufficiency, which is a pulling or tugging sensation in the muscle that occurs because you've put it in a position in which it cannot contract (such as occurs with your quadriceps in a hurdler's stretch), or you are essentially trying to pull the joint apart by its connective tissue—and that's not healthy.

While many folks may look back wistfully to a time in their younger days when they believed themselves to be "more flexible," because they could "execute a full side split," the reasoning behind such beliefs is faulty. We are no longer able to perform the impressive maneuvers that we could execute when we were younger because the capsules in the hip have now matured, and our femurs (upper-leg bones) have become bigger. With bigger bones, the movement potential in the hip capsule is now more restricted, as it should be to accommodate adult-size bones. Note that many martial artists who fanatically stretch are not immune from hip replacements and knee replacements as they age, which is a direct result of their attempting to force their joints into vulnerable positions. Similarly, children on sports teams are told to stretch all the time by their coaches, and many develop pulled groin muscles as a result.

Often adults who believe they have suffered a loss in flexibility have actually suffered a loss of functional strength. If they attempt to perform a full split, they won't make themselves any stronger, but, as with other such stretches, they may produce some improvement in their ability to perform this maneuver by virtue of both practicing and creating enough damage at the joint to allow it that degree of laxity. It is neither desirable nor necessary to do so to enhance your flexibility.

CARDIOVASCULAR STIMULATION

Virtually every study undertaken to assess the cardiovascular effects of proper strength training has concluded that they at least equal the effects of more conventional approaches such as running or other steady-state activity.[17] This makes sense, as your aerobic system is operational 24-7, not just when you take part in a weekly aerobics class or go for a run. It is simply involved to a greater degree whenever your muscles are made to perform work of a demanding nature.

Remember that the purpose of the cardiovascular system is to supply certain nutrients that are needed by the muscles and to help remove the by-products of the consumption and utilization of these nutrients. Cardiovascular health is often confused with aerobic conditioning, the latter of which is always specific to a particular activity, such as running or stationary cycling. Cardiovascular health, by contrast, equates to the ability of the heart, lungs, and bloodstream to supply whatever the muscles need. According to an abundance of studies, the cardiovascular system receives tremendous stimulation and benefit from resistance exercise.

RESISTANCE TRAINING: THE BEST KIND OF EXERCISE

A review of the more recent literature suggests that resistance training may be the best way to train the cardiovascular system. The only way to get at the cardiac or vascular system, after all, is by performing mechanical work with the muscles. It only makes sense that the higher the intensity and quality of the muscular work, the greater will be the effect on the systems that must support muscular work. Recall that, viewed in a biologic framework, exercise is an irritant stimulus that acts on the body (an organism); if the stimulus/intensity is high enough, and the organism has the available resources (rest and nutrition), it will produce an adaptive response. Ergo, raising the stimulus/intensity will produce a more pronounced and well-preserved adaptive response.

How do we know that resistance training produces a strong cardiovascular effect? A common misconception is that high muscular tension increases peripheral vascular resistance and traps venous blood, which inhibits venous return. These supposed effects would then act to decrease cardiac output. This theory makes little sense. Venous return is largely dependent on muscle contraction to move blood centrally. Forceful muscle contractions should enhance, not inhibit, cardiac return. Furthermore, the release of catecholamines during intense exercise causes gut vasoconstriction but stimulates vasodilation in the muscles, the net effect of which is to decrease peripheral resistance. Decreased peripheral resistance combined with enhanced venous return enhances cardiac output. In addition, increased end-diastolic pressure enhances coronary artery perfusion, making the performance of meaningful exercise possible even for people with coronary artery narrowing. (See Figure 5.1.)

Evidence for this association came in an article from the June 1999 issue of the *American Journal of Cardiology*, which reported on a group of researchers who used right heart catheterization to measure hemodynamic changes during high-intensity leg press exercise in patients with stable congestive heart failure. The measurements taken noted significant increases in heart rate, mean arterial blood pressure, diastolic pulmonary artery pressure, and cardiac index. Furthermore, there was a significant decrease in peripheral vascular resistance, along with an increased cardiac work index and left ventricular stroke work index, suggesting enhanced left ventricular function.[18]

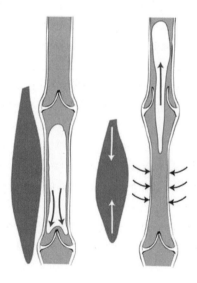

◼️| FIGURE 5.1.

Muscular contractions milk venous blood through one-way valves back toward the right side of the heart.

This study demonstrated that the assumptions people had formerly held about weight training's being dangerous for the heart were wrong. We had always been told that during weight training, the systemic vascular resistance was increased dramatically, so that the heart was now having to push against a lot more resistance, and that the blood was trapped in the working muscle. We were also told that cardiac return (the amount of blood returning to the heart) was diminished by weight training.

What we've since discovered is that the exact opposite is true: during high-intensity strength training, you're having dilation of the blood vessels in the peripheral musculature, which leads to a decrease in systemic vascular resistance. The squeezing of the contracting muscles is actually milking venous blood back to the heart. The amount of blood returned to the right side of the heart determines the amount of blood that is ejected from the left side of the heart, and the amount of blood ejected from the left side of the heart during systole determines the amount of blood that backwashes to the base of the aorta during diastole (in other words, the volume of blood that passively rushes into the coronary arteries, which originate at the base of the aorta). (See Figure 5.2.) Coronary artery blood flow is directly proportionate to venous return (the amount of blood coming back to the right side of the heart), as that volume determines the amount of blood ejected out of the left side of the heart, which, in turn, determines the amount of blood that washes into the base of the aorta. (See Figure 5.3.) So, strength training can be defined as a form of exercise that enhances coronary artery blood flow, and it does so by a means that decreases systemic vascular resistance.

With strength training, you're able to perform a type of exercise that enhances your coronary artery blood flow while simultaneously decreasing the amount of resistance against which your heart has to pump. The evidence is clear: strength training is a modality of exercise that is as safe and productive as possible from a cardiovascular standpoint. The American Heart Association has even included strength training as one of the major components of cardiac rehabilitation. The fact that it made this statement is an indicator of how powerful the evidence in favor of strength training is. It takes a considerable amount of objective data to get a conservative body to alter its position, as the AHA did in a scientific statement published

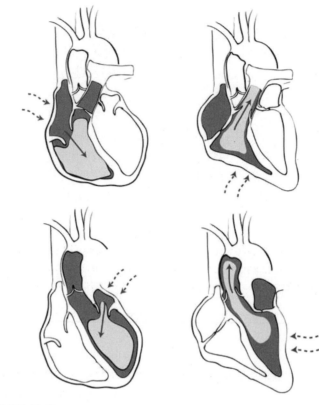

███ FIGURE 5.2.

Increased venous return from these intense muscular contractions results in a higher volume of blood moving through the heart.

August 2, 2007, in their journal *Circulation*. (The AHA had never embraced strength training before.)

Peripheral Effects

Beyond the undeniable effects on the cardiovascular system, resistance training has major impacts through peripheral adaptations, mainly in muscle strength. Doctors have routinely told their patients that just performing activities of daily life such as walking, taking the stairs, gardening, and yard work can help to preserve cardiovascular health. Unfortunately, the age-related loss of muscle (sarcopenia) can undermine people's ability

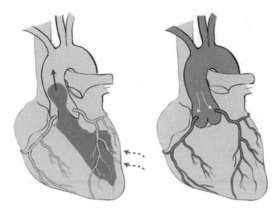

FIGURE 5.3.

The increased volume of blood ejected out of the aorta results in an increased volume of backwash during the cardiac relaxation cycle. This increased backwash results in increased blood flow into the coronary arteries, which originate at the base of the aorta.

to carry out those activities, but resistance training can prevent and even reverse sarcopenia.[19] Furthermore, as a muscle becomes stronger, fewer motor units will have to be recruited to perform a given task, thus reducing the demand on the cardiovascular system. Not only will a properly conducted strength-training program tax the musculature at a high level, and thus create a powerful cardiovascular stimulus, but also it will do so while simultaneously producing hemodynamic changes that minimize the risk of cardiac ischemia, producing the most profound peripheral changes in the form of muscle strengthening.[20]

THE BEST RESISTANCE-TRAINING PROGRAM

The best resistance-training program, then, would be one that is of high intensity but of low force, so that the beneficial effects of exercise can be obtained without the risk of injury. Heightened intensity is also helpful, as the duration of the workout must be shortened, which means that the recovery interval between exercise sessions can be prolonged. A brief and infrequent exercise protocol has been proved to go a long way toward improving long-term compliance with any exercise program.

At our facilities, we use a slower rate of lifting and lowering the weight—in some instances, a SuperSlow™ protocol, which involves lifting the resistance over a ten-second time span and lowering it over a ten-second time span. The excessively slow lifting speed provides two beneficial effects. First, by moving slowly, the weight cannot get moving under its own momentum, and this enhances muscular loading and intensifies the exercise. Second, the slow movement eliminates acceleration. Since force = mass × acceleration, we can greatly reduce the amount of force that the trainee will encounter.

The SuperSlow protocol was originally devised for use with osteoporosis patients.[21] It was so effective at raising intensity that workouts of about twelve minutes in length have proved to be optimal when coupled with a recovery interval of seven days for most subjects. We have been able to double subjects' strength in about twelve to twenty weeks. Research performed by Dr. Wayne Wescott compared the SuperSlow protocol with standard-repetition-speed resistance training and noted a 50 percent better strength gain in the SuperSlow group.[22] The researchers were so astounded that they later repeated the study and were able to reproduce the results.[23]

The workout described in Chapter 4, then, represents about as perfect an exercise program as could be desired. It accomplishes everything that we've outlined in a manner that other modalities cannot equal. It's also a program that has the broadest applicability. This is not to say that strength training alone will make you an exceptional track-and-field athlete. If you want a specific metabolic adaptation, you can produce it only by practicing that specific metabolic adaptation. If, for instance, you want to be good at the 100-yard dash and you want your metabolism to adapt specifically to that, then that's what you need to do. If, six months from now, there's a 10k coming up in which you want to run, then you must cultivate the skill set necessary to adapt specifically to that activity.

However, it is important to recognize that it is not necessary to run a 10k or take a yoga class or perform daily sessions on a treadmill, stationary bicycle, or elliptical to enhance your cardiovascular system—and being able to perform these activities will not make you healthier or cause you to live longer. Almost every form of exercise other than proper strength training carries with it a good chance of undermining your health because of the accumulated forces involved.

Obviously, proper strength training can significantly benefit both your health and your fitness levels, and it can do so in a way that will never be injurious or undermine your goals. Of course, you can continue to train conventionally in the hope that you will run a faster 10k or be able to compete in a marathon—and hope that your joints and connective tissue can survive your efforts. You can make the specific metabolic adaptations necessary to do well in all of these things, but, make no mistake, when those metabolic changes happen, they'll be happening in *muscle*.

Enhancing the Body's Response to Exercise

t often surprises people to learn that no amount of supplements, such as protein powders, vitamins, and minerals, will ever "stimulate" muscle growth. In a laboratory study conducted in 1975 by Harvard Medical School professor Alfred Goldberg, laboratory rats that were denied food of any sort produced unusual muscle growth—providing that their muscles were exercised intensely beforehand.[1] While it can be argued that this is interesting information for rats, the fact remains that mammalian muscle tissue was shown to grow under starvation conditions when it received a high-intensity stimulus to do so.

The first requisite, then, of doing everything you can to optimize the results of your workouts is not to run to your nearest health food store to stock up on the latest supplement du jour; it is instead to ensure that you are training with sufficient intensity to warrant your body's producing the desired adaptive response. Typically, whether the subject is a rodent or a human, if success has been achieved with this aspect of the process, growth will follow.

The exercise modality of the Big-Five baseline workout represents a phenomenal stimulus to your body. It is more than adequate for tripping the growth mechanism into motion. Once this has occurred, your body will produce an adaptive change in the form of bigger, stronger muscles and an enhancement of the metabolic systems that support them. This is a biologic process and, as with all biologic processes, requires time—up to seven days, on average. This "waiting" period can be frustrating for many people, particularly those who seek "instant" results. Muscle growth, alas, is not an instant process; it doesn't happen solely as a result of the application of

Heed the Need

Being an ER physician on a rotating schedule, I know that my response to a workout and my ability to recover from one workout to the next is largely dictated by where I am in my schedule. If it's a week in which I work two day shifts, two 5 P.M.–1 A.M. shifts, a pullback to 3 P.M.–11 P.M., and then another pullback to a day shift, followed by a night shift, my recovery will be poor. This poor-recovery factor needs to be taken into account.

A regular sleep cycle in which you're getting seven to eight hours of sleep per night is an enormous help for enhancing recovery and your body's response to the exercise stimulus. I think that's simply because the hormones that we use to deal with stress, particularly cortisol, are released in a specific diurnal cycle that peaks at approximately 2 P.M.–3 P.M. and then again in the wee hours of the morning. That 2 P.M.–3 P.M. dip in cortisol explains why a lot of European countries have a siesta, or naptime, during that period of the day, in which pretty much everything shuts down. When you're able to pay heed to those natural needs of the body, you're going to enhance your ability to recover from the exercise stimulus.

—Doug McGuff, M.D.

the appropriate training stimulus. It is a consequence of the application of the appropriate stimulus and the passage of sufficient time. If insufficient time is allotted for the body to produce the response that the high-intensity workout stimulated, then the body simply will fail to do so. Likewise, if the workout stimulus was too low in intensity to trigger the growth mechanism of the body into motion, then you can wait for an infinity of eternities, and nothing will be produced.

Nevertheless, many trainees fret that they are "not doing enough" while waiting out the necessary time before the next workout can be performed. They are fretting needlessly, because the best thing that trainees can do during their off time is to tend to the needs of the body, ensuring that it is fully capable of delivering the requested response.

Sufficient rest

To help your body in its attempts to produce the desired response from training, it is important to ensure that it is sufficiently recuperated, and one of the biggest aids to recuperation after an intense workout is adequate sleep.[2] It is during sleep that the body recovers, when it relaxes and when its repair processes can proceed without interruption.

Adequate hydration

Being well hydrated helps your body in many ways. Apart from the fact that muscle is composed of roughly 76 percent water, adequate hydration maximizes your circulating blood volume. This benefit, in turn, maximizes the delivery of nutrients to recovering muscles while withdrawing waste products that accrue as a result of intense muscular contractions. Studies performed on subjects who strength-trained and on athletes have conclusively established that proper hydration aids significantly in optimizing recovery and enhancing muscular performance.[3]

The importance of adequate hydration is seen daily in emergency rooms throughout the world, particularly with elderly patients, whose thirst mechanism is often impeded. A common tipping point in their becoming ill is inadequate hydration, which impedes the ability of the bloodstream to deliver sufficient oxygen to the tissues. Dehydration results in a constriction of blood volume to the point where they can no longer perfuse their tissues with sufficient oxygen, causing them to become acidotic. Once this happens, the metabolism becomes almost entirely glycolytic, producing lactic acid. At the same time, a consequence of acidosis is a drop in blood pressure, resulting in acute sickness. Many such elderly patients who arrive at emergency rooms from a local nursing home look as if they are dying, but after the attending physician administers a liter of IV fluid over the course of two to three hours, they awake, completely alert, and appear completely well.

Another important side benefit of proper hydration is that your body's adaptation to the resistance-training stimulus effects some degree of adaptation that is largely hormonal.[4] Any hormonal effect is very much dependent on that hormone's being circulated to the appropriate receptor sites.

As illustrated in Figure 6.1, the wall of any cell in the body comprises what is called a phospholipid bilayer. This bilayer is made up of fatty acids that have both a head portion, which is water attracting, and a tail portion, which is water repelling. Every cell membrane envelops the contents of the cell. Both the interior and exterior of the cell are water based. The water-attracting heads face outward toward the extracellular fluid but also inward toward the intracellular fluid. This is accomplished by the two ends of the water-repelling tails facing each other in the interior of the cell wall. As a consequence, the receptor sites for hormones become sandwiched inside the interior of the cell wall in such a way that they protrude toward the interior and the exterior (depending on what they're interacting with) of the cell.

If you are well hydrated, the hormones are circulated to the necessary receptor sites for optimal response. In addition, the cytoplasm (the water-containing interior of the cell) is maximally hydrated, which means that these same receptors, sitting as they do on the surface of the cell membrane, become maximally convexed into the environment where the hormones are circulating, thus allowing for maximal hormonal interaction with the receptor sites. If you are dehydrated, though, these same cells become somewhat concaved, because the cytoplasm is not fully hydrated. A lot of the receptors that sit on the edge of the cell membrane now involute away from the external environment where the circulating hormones can interact with them, thus preventing all of the hormonal responses necessary to produce an optimal anabolic response to the stimulus.

The act of hydration, as can be seen, enhances the hormonal responsiveness of the body after the exercise stimulus has been applied. Not only

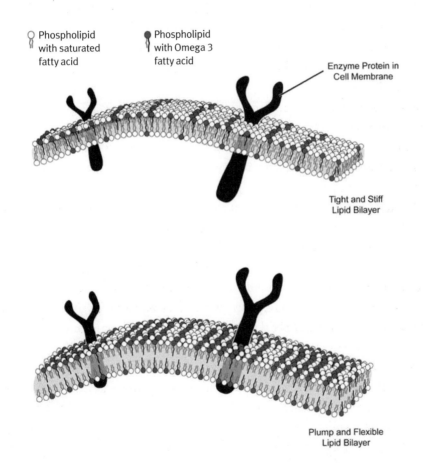

FIGURE 6.1.

Increased hydration pushes the cell membrane outward, which increases the exposure of the hormone receptors on the cell. Increased omega-3 fatty acids promote a plumper cell membrane, further enhancing hormone receptor exposure.

does hydration allow the body to more effectively circulate hormones, but also, because the cells have been, in effect, plumped up, the receptor sites are now pushed toward the exterior of the cell wall, where they can better interact with the circulating hormones.

One hormone that is released in greater quantities into the general circulation as a result of the training stimulus is the stress hormone cortisol, as noted earlier. The recovery process of the body requires that cortisol be modulated, with noninflammatory hormones and chemical messengers predominating during the recovery period. (This is another instance of catabolism and anabolism.) Cortisol is produced in the middle layer of the adrenal gland, which is layered out in three sectors:

1. The mineralocorticoids
2. The corticosteroids
3. The sex hormones

Aldosterone and the antidiuretic hormones are located in the outermost layer of the adrenal gland, with cortisol just underneath them, but the boundary between these two layers is not necessarily sharp. If you should become dehydrated, you will need to activate the adrenal glands to produce more hormone, which facilitates fluid retention. Your body will then be stimulated to secrete more aldosterone and antidiuretic hormone—and dragged along with these will be cortisol. That is, these substances are so close in the structure of the adrenal gland that the stress hormones will be released more aggressively if you're not adequately hydrated. Adequate hydration, therefore, plays a lead role in the hormonal component of the recovery process.

How much water should one drink to help the recovery process? A good rule of thumb for proper hydration is to consume roughly three liters per day.

ADEQUATE NUTRITION

Adequate—but not excessive—nutrition is another contributor to optimizing the body's response to the exercise stimulus. Excessive nutrition in the form of calories from food will only make you fat. The same situation exists with calories contained in supplements, along with the additional problem that many supplements have proved to be stressful to the body. A well-balanced diet, as opposed to supplementation, is important because it allows you to obtain the necessary nutritional components that aid in the recovery of the body after a workout and that provide the elements to build additional muscle during the growth production that follows. More important, a well-balanced diet does so within the natural-food matrix for which these nutrients were intended.

We may be able to isolate certain vitamins that, in isolation, may have beneficial effects, but it is still better to consume them when they are contained in the food matrix where they originate, as an infinite number of potential cofactors that result in their being beneficial to health can be lost in the isolation process. When a vitamin or mineral is removed from the environment it shares with other healthful cofactors (such as the apple in which the vitamin C molecule is contained), isolating it may not necessarily be helpful at all and may even result in a burden that the body then must ameliorate, thus delaying the recovery process to some degree. This aspect of nutritional science is not yet fully understood, including by the manufacturers of nutritional supplements. For the moment, Mother Nature still has the upper hand.

PUTTING STRESSORS INTO PERSPECTIVE

One of the most worthwhile steps a trainee can take to create a better metabolic environment in which to build muscle is to keep other life stressors to a minimum. This aspect often is not within people's control, but as much as it may be, it's advisable to opt for a lower-stress approach to life. In modern society, citizens frequently do not modulate their responses appropriately. Small stressors ("I'm going to be late in picking my kids up from hockey practice") are allowed to assume much larger importance than they merit, even rising to the level of inciting a fight-or-flight response. From an evolutionary standpoint, such a response would ordinarily be evoked only in times of physical attack or life-threatening situations. For these reasons and more, it behooves you to learn to treat mundane stressors as the minor events they are and to react to them appropriately, rather than disproportionately.

DON'T CULTIVATE TRAINING ANGST

During your "off" days, always remember that your purpose in training is to enhance your functional ability. This requires you to have recovered sufficiently between workouts so that you end up spending more time above baseline (the strength level that you had prior to your workout) than below. To enjoy the advantages gained through resistance training, you want those advantages present for several days, rather than just for a few hours of one day. Otherwise, what exactly is the benefit? What, for instance, would be the point of taking six steps backward in order to take one step forward?

The immediate consequence of a proper strength-training workout is that the trainee gets weaker—and remains so for several days while the body replenishes the energy debt it incurred. Only once this has taken place will the body start to produce the adaptive response (i.e., growth). During the first four to six days after a workout, you are technically below baseline. The ideal is to train in such a way that allows enough recovery to take place so that you are spending more time during a given week above baseline than below baseline.

What needs to be cultivated is an antidote to the neurosis exhibited by those trainees who live to "get back into the gym and train." Presumably, you want to get the most that is possible from your exercise program, which, by definition, means that you want to be in the supranormal state for at least as long as you've been in the subnormal state, in order to feel as though you at least broke even. Remember, you're not going to "lose" anything by extending your recovery period to eight, nine, ten, or even fourteen days. A workout, per se, makes you weaker—it drops your physiology below baseline. So, what is the upside to performing more workouts than are required and that only exacerbate this negative purpose? Answer: None.

Knowing this, attempt to maintain a generally relaxed state of mind such that you're not worrying about the workout and recovery process. Ignore the fitness magazines whose sole purpose for existing is to sell you supplements and instill a sense of training angst by convincing you that you're not doing enough.

All of the aforementioned advice optimally sets the stage for your body to amass the necessary resources to make its adaptive response as stimulated by the workout. Remember that you're asking your body to make an investment in a tissue that it considers metabolically expensive. If any of these vital points is unaddressed, the reservation of resources for the building of more muscle tissue will inevitably be withheld.

In summary, enhancing the body's response to exercise consists of paying attention to what are in reality basic principles. But never underestimate the power of paying attention to the basics in promoting the numbers on the recovery side of the equation.

Tweaking the Exercise Stimulus

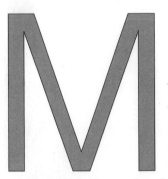uscle growth is a multifactorial process that is an offshoot of muscular contraction against a progressively increasing load over time. With inroad as the standard, several contributing factors are brought into play, including the momentary weakening of muscle, the accumulated by-products of fatigue (such as lactic acid), an increase in the load against which the muscles are made to contract, and microtrauma to tissue that facilitates the process of repair and growth. All of these factors contribute to the growth process, and with the inroad modality, their contributions are more or less even. The result is an excellent balance of factors that effectively combine to stimulate a positive change in the body.

As discussed, to qualify as productive exercise, training has to be demanding (of high intensity) to the muscles but performed in such a way that force is controlled and the muscles are being weakened to a point of positive failure. This quality can be said to represent the hub of the wheel,

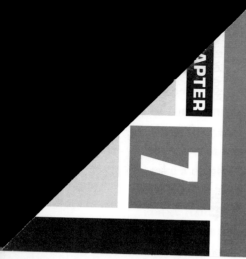

...okes that extend out to represent the various components ... However, caution must be the trainee's byword during ...e thing we have learned over many years of training cli-...ring off the hub to pursue one of the "spokes" seems to ...ionate toll on recovery. This caution particularly applies ...n as SuperSlow that emphasize a deep inroad—in which a ...n the volume and frequency of training is going to require ...ds of recovery for the body to replenish its energy reserves ...adaptive response.

Muscle growth is the end result of several complex processes that cannot be infinitely reduced down to a single element. The various segments to which many people have attempted to reduce exercise over the years are now recognized as being merely the products of a multicomponent process that, in aggregate, produce a positive stimulus to the body. While micro-trauma, or damage to muscle tissue, is a known component of this stimulus process, that doesn't mean that damage, per se, should become the objective of a workout. You wouldn't, for instance, beat your quadriceps with a hammer until there is damage and expect to produce a benefit from this action. The benefit from exercise is produced within a specific context, and it's a context that is always multifactorial and complex. Not every cause produces a proportionate effect.

The Big-Five routine introduced in Chapter 4 will serve you as a reliable baseline program for building overall muscular size and strength throughout your training career. The reason it is so effective is that it produces a stimulus that permits all of the multifactorial components to come to bear on the body. Its touchstones are significant loading combined with a high intensity of effort. These two factors allow the trainee's muscles to contract and extend against that load until they are genuinely unable to continue doing so.

Among the many factors that combine to produce a strong stimulus to the body is an inroading process, which produces a significant amount of accumulated by-products of fatigue as well as microdamage to the muscular tissue. In addition, there is a transient loss of blood flow and oxygen delivery, followed by increased blood and oxygen delivery (known as "hyperemia"). Certain hormonal responses also are produced, but these, again, are secondary to the primary components of a significant load combined with intentional effort—two factors that produce all of the by-products of the stimulus that trainees desire from exercise.

The Big Five is a protocol that has a scientifically validated track record of success. Nevertheless, as you progress in strength, this basic, whole-body training protocol will at some point stop stimulating a positive adaptive response from your body. This occurs for two reasons. First, you will eventually come up against certain mechanical limitations in the equipment that are roadblocks to reaching the trigger point that will stimulate another round of increases in strength and muscle mass. Second, the accumulated workload of the existing program will eventually grow to the point where you can no longer recover from a workout in the span of seven days. This chapter will examine these impediments to future progress, as well as what remedies can be applied to overcome them.

We want to guard against prescribing any particular strength-training protocol, because there are multiple factors to the stimulus, and as you progress and improve, the degree of importance of different components may change. Sometimes, to get more of one component of the stimulus, you will have to sacrifice another component to some extent. This negotiation is accomplished by cycling between different protocols that emphasize different components of the stimulus, in order to obtain maximal benefit from your workouts over the course of your training career.

For instance, if your intention is to push your aerobic system harder through accumulated lactic acid as a result of greater fatigue, you may have to sacrifice load to some degree in favor of slightly more time spent against somewhat lighter resistance. The converse would be to emphasize load by performing a protocol that involves heavier weights (such as negative-only or Max Contraction), in which each rep can last as little as five seconds, sacrificing the accumulated by-products of fatigue to some extent. These variations will not represent permanent changes, mind you. They are simply deviations from the baseline program that will serve to optimize or tweak the training stimulus and, depending on your genetics, your response to exercise.

ROADBLOCK—EXCESSIVE INTENSITY

A good many trainees, particularly within high-intensity training circles, infer that if high-intensity muscular contraction is the key factor required to stimulate the body to produce growth, it follows that if one could somehow devise a "superintensity" training technique, one would be able to stimulate the body into producing "super" results. Indeed, this is the logic underlying all so-called "advanced" training techniques. This inference is not completely wrong, but it certainly is a half-baked concept.

For one thing, it may not be necessary. As trainees grow stronger, the intensity of their muscular contractions increases as a matter of course, because they are now contracting their muscles against heavier weights. For another, drastically upping the stress applied to the body's musculature through a "superintense" training technique places a much greater demand on the body's energy-recovery system. This could set up a situation in which a recovery and overcompensation process that might have been completed in seven to twelve days now will require several months.[1]

An old proverb cautions, "The perfect is the destroyer of the good." This warning has a direct application to trainees' desire to expose their muscles to the "ultimate" stimulus in the belief that they will thereby force their bodies to produce the ultimate in muscular development. When this belief manifests, it is imperative to ensure that science is not discarded in the pursuit of glossy images of physical perfection. Trainees' frustration is understandable and might be stated as, "I've worked out so hard, I've trained in a high-intensity fashion for months, but my body hasn't produced the gains in muscle mass that I hoped for." They perceive a gulf between what they want and what their bodies are capable of producing. The former is dictated by desire, the latter by genetics.

Since genetics has rained on desire's parade, it is discounted or otherwise ignored as the trainee ventures off in search of a magic bullet. Training intensity is then dialed up to phenomenally high levels, involving greater energy expenditures and increased musculature microtrauma. When results are not forthcoming from this attack, the frequency of the application of the training stress is increased—again, all in the belief that the body can be forced to respond. The only thing being forced, meanwhile, is a deeper catabolic state from which it could now take months to recover.

Of course, it is a somewhat natural inclination for a trainee to associate the intensity level of exercise with the benefit sought: the muscles must be made to work at a certain threshold level of intensity to stimulate the body to produce any benefit at all. The fallacy is that it does not follow that going well beyond this level of intensity brings any additional benefit whatsoever. The concept of the narrow therapeutic window is always in effect, reminding us that too much of a good thing is decidedly negative—whether it's intensity or volume (which, to some degree, equate to the same thing in regard to putting a drain on the body's limited reserve of resources).

It's the same faulty reasoning that leads people to overdose on their medications: "The directions say to take two tablets every four hours, but since I really want this headache to be gone as fast as possible, I'll take four to five tablets every two hours." Such thought put into action does not stimulate more of the desired positive response; instead, it sets into motion a crisis situation whereby the body can't cope with what it has been given. It's akin to believing that to enhance your suntan, you've got to "take it to the next level" by exposing your skin to the highest possible level of UV radiation. This tactic won't produce a better tan, but it will gain you admittance to a hospital emergency room for third-degree burns.

The typical sources of training information are guilty of promulgating the notion that a supranormal stimulus (a stimulus beyond what is currently being employed) is always going to result in a much greater compensatory response. Just as with volume and frequency, intensity has a threshold; pushing beyond it doesn't necessarily get you better results and can easily leave you worse off.

More Isn't Better

I t bears repeating that the arguments that have been made in high-intensity circles that high intensity is the common denominator of what is producing results, and therefore, the higher the intensity, the better the results, are fallacious. It doesn't follow that if something is true, then having even more of it makes it *truer*. You can't go down that slippery slope.

For instance, there is a high-intensity training protocol called "hyper reps," which involves performing a maximum-effort lifting of the weight followed immediately by a maximum-effort lowering of the weight. This is typically carried on until the trainee becomes too weak to lift even the movement arm of the machine. This is an intense protocol, and in some instances—if applied sparingly—it can make a difference for some poor responders. However, almost universally, particularly in myself, I find that it's a level of inroad, fatigue, and damage from which the body is not able to adequately recover. If I just go to positive failure, I get better results. Similarly, SuperSlow was big on the "deep inroad technique," which was to continue to push on the movement arm until you couldn't sustain the movement arm at all. (You would, for instance, be in the bottom position and just continue to push statically until you could not even keep your limb in contact with the mechanism.) What I found was that my results were always better if I just stopped right at positive failure and didn't do that ten-second or fifteen-second (or even thirty-second) push beyond. That extra effort resulted in no additional benefit and severely compromised my recovery. It was too much.

—Doug McGuff, M.D.

- -

When you are training, you must have a clear understanding of the purpose of the protocols introduced in this chapter, including what they will do and, more important, what they won't do. If you have grown stronger, it's essential to pay attention to your recovery ability during the periods in which you employ any of these protocols. They are not a means of trying to increase the stimulus, with the assumption that in so doing, you will surely stimulate a proportionate increase in body response. Our experience tells us otherwise. If careful attention isn't paid to reducing the volume and frequency in conjunction with the employment of such techniques, no response will be possible.

OBSTACLE NUMBER ONE: MECHANICAL STICKING POINTS

Depending on the equipment a trainee is using, certain mechanical impediments could stand in the way of inroading deeply enough to stimulate an optimal response. In the course of our own training and in supervising the training of others, we have noted that a lot of what we are calling "advanced" techniques are not performed foremost with the intention of tweaking the stimulus for better results. Rather, they are being executed to counter the problem of the trainees' having developed a level of strength that is incompatible with the equipment at hand. This problem typically concerns incongruities in strength curve and/or leverage that make continued progress difficult.

Let's say, by way of illustration, that you're exercising on a leg press machine, and there is a mismatch between the cam profile of the equipment and the force output of your leg muscles. This type of scenario is often referred to as a mechanical sticking point. Here, the sticking point can be attributable to a combination of the machine's cam profile (which on many machines simply isn't accurate, resulting in too much resistance being applied to a muscle when it is least capable of handling it—as discussed in Chapter 4) and your joint angle as you come out of the bottom position of the leg press, where you have minimal leverage. This mechanical "speed bump" now has to be overcome in the range of motion of the exercise. When a trainee is first attempting an exercise and has a factor of strength that is X, overcoming this obstacle can be likened to having to push a Yugo over that speed bump. If, over a span of time, the strength of that same trainee is compounded to X^2 or X^3 on that same piece of equipment, a much heavier weight now must be pushed over that bump, transforming the little Yugo into a Mack truck.

Once a trainee has reached this level of strength, merely continuing to perform the same dynamic protocol may actually prevent any progression of resistance. Instead, what the trainee requires at this juncture is a continued stimulus that trumps the mechanical inefficiencies of the equipment so that the speed bump can be successfully finessed and progress can resume.

The upcoming sections survey some protocols that can assist you at this stage of your development.

Segmented Manual Assistance (Forced Repetitions)

In the early stages of impasse, trainees can use segmented manual assistance to get over a speed bump, thus allowing for the completion of another full repetition in such a manner that their time under load will stay within the realm that produces the optimal stimulus. A study that tested the effectiveness of segmented manual assistance led the experimenters to conclude:

> The forced repetition exercise system induced greater acute hormonal and neuromuscular responses than a traditional maximum repetition exercise system and therefore may be used to manipulate acute resistance exercise variables in athletes.[2]

To perform segmented manual assistance, once you cannot move the resistance, your training partner or trainer diminishes a portion of the load by either lifting the machine's movement arm or pressing on your limbs with just enough force to allow you to get past the sticking point, and then easing off so that you are allowed to perform the remainder of the movement on your own. Performing one or two such segmented manual assistance repetitions is sufficient.

Partial Repetitions

Partial repetitions can be performed to good effect on either side of the speed bump. If you choose to perform them on the side closer to full contraction (in the leg press, this would be the position in which your legs are moving closer to being fully locked out), you can and should use more weight, as you will no longer be limited in how much weight you can use through your weakest point in the range of motion—the sticking point. This strategy will accustom your muscles to more intense muscular contractions and to producing more force, as is necessary to contract against a heavier weight. This action can be just what is required to move you over the speed bump when you return to full-range training. Similarly, the partial repetition can be performed in your weakest position, allowing you to focus and strengthen the range leading up to the sticking point, which will also give you more strength in an area that sorely requires it.

Don't worry that performing exercises in a limited range of motion will somehow compromise your strength in performing full-range exercise. In a study conducted at the University of Southern Mississippi comparing full-range-of-motion resistance exercise with partial-range-of-motion exercise, the researchers found that lifting weights through a partial range of motion developed strength equally as effectively as exercising muscles through a full range of motion. They concluded: "These findings appear to suggest that partial range of motion training can positively influence the development of maximal strength."[3]

Prior to this study, it had been believed that muscle strength improves only at the joint angle at which it is trained and that if you didn't train with a full range of motion of a joint, you would have weakness in the joint angles that weren't trained. It was also believed that performing only the second half of the lift (from the sticking point up to lockout, not returning to the full starting position) would not improve the trainee's strength at the start of the lift. This study revealed that this was an unfounded belief, as strength increases were the same for the partial-range-of-motion group as they were for the full-range-of-motion group.

This finding makes sense, as exercising throughout a full range of motion has never been established as the sine qua non of joint health. Joints are intrinsically healthy as long as they don't encounter the kind of cross-repetitive forces that are going to cause damage to them—either loss of articular cartilage or development of osteophytes as a result of chronic, recurrent damaging force. If these conditions are absent, the trainee will maintain normal joint health as long as the surrounding supporting musculature is strong enough to continue to move the limbs around the joint.

Timed Static Hold

If you perform a timed static contraction at the point and location of the speed bump, which is also typically the point where positive failure occurs, you can achieve a deeper inroad into your starting level of strength. The timed static contraction can be performed either right on top of the speed bump, if that is where you desire, or after you have performed the maximal number of repetitions that you are capable of completing through that sticking point. At the point where you can no longer complete another full repetition, simply perform a static hold in this position for as long as you can, until you begin to be pulled back down through the negative portion of the movement. Only one such timed static hold is required and should be sustained for approximately ten seconds.

Rest-Pause

Another technique that can help with sticking points is the protocol of rest-pause. This time-honored strength-training technique was rediscovered and refined to a large measure during the late 1970s by former bodybuilding champion Mike Mentzer. The way we advocate performing the technique is to take your set to a point of positive failure—the point at which another full repetition isn't possible—and pause for a brief rest (five to ten seconds) until you are able to just complete another repetition.

The number of rest-pause reps that you might perform will depend on the movement and on your fiber-type expression in that movement. For instance, if you're reaching failure in seventy seconds or seventy-five seconds, that would indicate that the muscle groups you are training have a predominantly fast-twitch profile. In such a case, the rest-pause will have to be longer, because the fast-twitch motor units take longer to recover. You may have to wait as long as fifteen to thirty seconds before attempting your next repetition, to be able to complete it.

Typically, only one rest-pause repetition is adequate. However, if it takes you 90 to 120 seconds of time under load during your set before you reach failure, the rest-pause can be as short as 5 seconds before you're ready to perform your next repetition. This time frame is more indicative of a slower-twitch muscular profile, and these (as we've seen) are faster-recovering fibers. Therefore, with this fiber-type profile, as many as three repetitions could be performed in rest-pause fashion without the risk of overtraining.

Rest-pause repetitions allow you a second round of recruiting the higher-order motor units without the necessity of going through all of the mechanical work leading up to the failure point.

Negative-Only

Another means of getting past a sticking point is to perform negative-only repetitions. Here the actual lifting, or positive, portion of the repetition is eliminated, so the trainee focuses solely on the lowering, or negative, portion. Studies have indicated that a tremendous amount of strength can be stimulated with such a protocol.[4] An added benefit is that the load and damage components of the stimulus receive the majority of the attention.

When performing negative-only exercise, "going to failure" refers to form failure—when you can no longer lower the resistance in five seconds—as opposed to taking the set to the point where you can no longer control the lowering of the weight. You lower the resistance as slowly as possible, but the set is complete when the resistance can no longer be lowered in five seconds (because you have grown so weak that the lowering now takes place in four seconds or less).

There was a day when trainees were told to continue beyond this point and to keep attempting to lower the resistance until no downward control was possible and the weight simply came crashing down. We believe this procedure to be downright dangerous. A safe form of failure needs to be defined, and if the benefit from negative-only training is to be found in the increased-load component of the exercise, then it should be obtainable within a reasonable amount of form failure.

Remember that all of these techniques are a means of continuing to proceed with an exercise that, owing to mechanical limitations, has ceased being an effective stimulus for positive change.

OBSTACLE NUMBER TWO: THE NARROW THERAPEUTIC WINDOW REVISITED

Chapter 3 introduced the concept of the "narrow therapeutic window;" the phenomenon in which the therapeutic effect of a certain exercise or exercise program levels out, but its toxic effect continues to rise. This, contrary to popular opinion in fitness circles, occurs not because the program is no longer effective but rather because it is now so effective that training once every seven days is no longer a sufficient dosing frequency to allow for recovery and adaptation. No matter how intense or perfectly delivered the exercise stimulus is, if the body is not adequately recovered, no adaptive response will be made.

The major factor that erodes recovery ability is the total accumulated workload encountered in a given workout. When you first begin working out, you are too weak to accumulate a workload that will exceed your recovery ability, but within six to twelve weeks of training, you will become strong enough to exceed your recovery ability, and your progress will halt.

What follows is an oversimplification, but it will suit our purpose. Let us assume that under ideal circumstances, your recovery ability can accommodate 12,000 foot-pounds of work in a one-week period. Initially, you might be able to produce about 8,000 foot-pounds of work per workout, and thus you are easily able to produce results from one weekly workout. As you get stronger, however, you can now produce 13,000 foot-pounds of work in the same number of exercises as when you began. Consequently, you have performed more work than you can now recover from in a seven-day period.

Both of our fitness facilities double as ongoing research laboratories. We learn something from every client we train, and we have gained specific insight on matters such as how infrequently one can train before the process breaks down, how intense the exercise stimulus needs to be, and whether advanced trainees benefit more (or less) from training with increased intensity. We have experimented with increasing and decreasing the volume of the workouts and have also noted the effects of the workout stimulus and training frequency on clients who are experiencing an increase in daily life stressors. All of that data has been educational, and some has been fascinating.

We've learned, for instance, that some trainees can stop training entirely for up to three months and still hold on to the positive adaptive response they obtained from their last workout. (They actually return to their training stronger than they were when they stopped training three months previously.) Despite these knowledge strides, there is still a lot of gray in the realm of training frequency. We know that training once a week is sufficient for the body to produce a desirable response from the workout stimulus, but we don't yet know if training once every two weeks (as the subject grows stronger) or using just one set per week might not allow the body to produce even better results. So, we don't yet know with exactitude how long the window of opportunity stays open for the average client from when the gain shows up until it goes away, but the evidence we're amassing suggests that, in a lot of cases, it doesn't have to be a defined period.

It certainly has to be a *minimal* period, but once that minimal period has been passed, the additional amount of time that elapses can be highly variable and may not prove to be a negative experience for the trainee. Sometimes an individual will work out once every seven to ten days for a protracted period, but then something happens in the person's life, and he or she will average working out only once every two or three weeks for a span of months, at which point the trainee will return to the once-every-seven-to-ten-days frequency—with no ill effects. This irregularity may even be necessary for optimal production of workout benefits and for the health of the organism, given that humans evolved out of a chaotic, irregular existence and that chaotic irregularity is what defines the body's adaptive capabilities.

Sometimes the attempt to reduce such an adaptive biologic process to simple algebra is not the answer. As long as a certain minimum recovery interval is obtained, there may be, of necessity, some variation in the work-out scheduling. Some ebb and flow is probably desirable, because while some components may be quick in recovering, there may be small components that are not so quick and that can benefit from periods of extended laying off from the training stress.

For instance, the biggest glycogen stores are in the fastest-twitch motor units, but those high-order fast-twitch motor units evolved and adapted for high-intensity emergency events, which occur relatively infrequently. These motor units are what get tapped when the car jack falls, and Grandma lifts the car off of Grandpa. Once they've been tapped, their recovery period is long. There are even faster units than just Types IIA, IIAB, and IIB, as outlined in Chapter 3. There's also a Type IIx motor unit, which is more predominant in sprinters who lack the alpha-actinin-3 gene (more on this in the following chapter), and the recovery interval for these is exceedingly prolonged.

An article in the September 2000 issue of *Scientific American* entitled "Muscle Genes and Athletic Performance," by Jesper L. Anderson, Peter Schjerling, and Bengt Saltin, noted that a lot of champion sprinters break world records when, for injury reasons, they have had to lay off high-intensity training in their sport for as long as three months. During that layoff, they did minimal work to maintain their skills but didn't do anything of a high-intensity nature, because of their injury—and that's when these world records occur, because these very-high-order motor units finally had time to recover. The authors of the article stated:

> The fast IIx myosin declined as expected during resistance training. But when training stopped, rather than simply returning to the pretraining level, the relative amount of IIx roughly doubled three months into detraining. So what does this mean for the sprinter, to whom IIx is crucial? Provide a period of reduced training before a competition.

As you get stronger, the problem becomes providing adequate work for all of your major muscle groups without exceeding your body's recovery ability. Often, by either inserting additional recovery days into your program or removing one or two compound exercises and replacing them with single-joint axis movements (isolation exercises), the training can be brought more in line with recovery ability.

Reducing the Big Five to a Big Three

One way to alter a workout program is by creating a Workout 1 and Workout 2 that divide the Big-Five exercises into two separate workouts, while salting in some isolation movements, which are introduced later in this chapter. Such a program might be set up as follows:

Workout 1
1. Pulldown
2. Chest press
3. Leg press

Workout 2
1. Seated row
2. Overhead press
3. Standing calf raise

Each workout would be performed in an alternating fashion, with seven days of rest between workouts. If progress should again slow, the trainee simply needs to insert additional rest days between workouts. There's no need for concern if the time "off" between workouts stretches out to ten to fourteen days. As discussed previously, these aren't really "off" days; they are days that the body now requires to replenish the energy reserves that were exhausted by the previous workout and to produce the growth that these workouts stimulated.

The Split Routine

Another means of accomplishing the same end is to divide the Big-Five exercises into three separate workouts to be performed on a rotating basis. This allows for the insertion of a few more single-axis movements into a program without incurring the risk of overtraining. Such workouts might be constructed along the following lines:

Workout 1 (chest, shoulders, and triceps)
1. Chest press
2. Lateral raise
3. Triceps pressdown

Workout 2 (legs and abdominals)
1. Leg press
2. Standing calf raise
3. Abdominal machine

Workout 3 (back and biceps)
1. Pulldown
2. Seated row
3. Shrug or lower back machine
4. Biceps curl

As with the previous scenario, each workout would be performed on an alternating basis, with seven days of rest in between. Once again, don't worry that each major muscle group is receiving direct stimulation only once every twenty-one days. There is sufficient overlapping of muscle groups to at least maintain the growth in between direct workout sessions, and we can attest that energy output and recovery ability, particularly recovery of the fast-twitch motor units, will necessitate longer spans of recovery time.

To attempt to quantify the energy output that the baseline workout exacts, let's give it a numeric value of 100 units of energy. As the trainee grows bigger and stronger, around 120 units of energy would be outputted throughout the whole body as the workout forces muscles to overcompensate and store more units of energy for use. Consequently, the seven days that once proved sufficient time for the body to recoup 100 units of energy will no longer be sufficient time to recoup 120 units of energy. A three-way split routine will provide an extra window of opportunity for the energy systems of the body to fully recover and overcompensate.

Single-Joint (Isolation) Exercises

If a modification needs to be made in your program to keep your workouts in line with your recovery ability, the following exercises can be substituted or incorporated into your workouts.

Standing Calf Raise. Standing calf raises can be performed either on a standing calf raise machine or on a block that is high enough that when your heels are fully extended, or stretched, they don't hit the floor. If using a standing calf raise machine, place your shoulders under the pads and your hands on the handles, and step onto the small block or platform. Making sure to keep your back straight, straighten your legs until they are locked straight (which they have to be to fully engage the gastrocnemius muscle). Keeping your legs locked straight, slowly raise your heels as high as they can go. Pause briefly in this position of full muscular contraction, and then lower your heels slowly until they are as low as you can stretch them. Don't pause in this bottom position, but slowly press into the platform with the balls of your feet, causing your heels to rise again to a position of full contraction. Repeat for your TUL.

If you are using free weights, take hold of a dumbbell in one hand, and step onto a raised block. Make certain that the block is solid and isn't going to tip over on you.

If you are holding the dumbbell in your right hand, you will be emphasizing the left calf, so remove your right leg (you can rest your right foot on your left heel), and balance on your left leg. Making sure to keep your left leg straight, contract your left calf until the heel is up as high as it can go. Pause briefly, and then lower your left heel, stretching out the calf as much as possible. Now slowly rise up again to a fully contracted position. Repeat for your TUL.

When you have finished training your left calf, transfer the dumbbell to your left hand and draw your left foot off the platform so that you can repeat the process with your right calf. Again, repeat for your TUL.

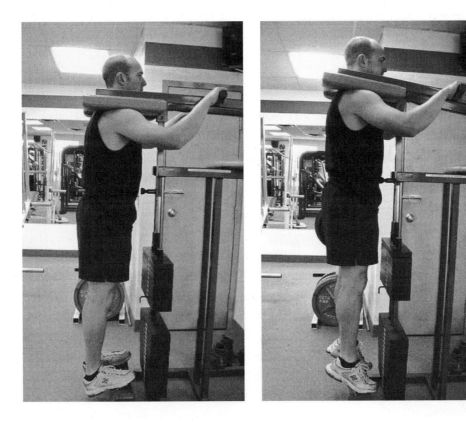

Standing calf raise (start and finish position)

Lateral Raise. Lateral raises can be performed either on a machine or with dumbbells. If using a machine, sit with your back on the pad. Make sure that the center of your shoulder joint is aligned with the center of the cam. Take hold of the handles so that your elbows are drawn back behind your body slightly and your upper arms are resting on the arm pads. Slowly lift your upper arms out to the sides until they are slightly above 90 degrees relative to your torso. Pause briefly in this fully contracted position, and then lower your arms slowly back to the starting position. Do not pause at the bottom, but slowly reverse direction and lift your arms back up to the point where your deltoids (specifically, the lateral head of the deltoid musculature) are fully contracted. Repeat for your TUL.

If using dumbbells, take hold of a dumbbell in each hand, and stand up straight. With a minimal bend in your elbows (so as not to strain your elbow joint), slowly draw your upper arms up to a point where they are slightly above 90 degrees relative to your torso. Pause briefly in this fully contracted position, and then lower the dumbbells slowly and under control back to the starting position. Again, do not rest in this position, but slowly reverse direction until your upper arms are again at or above the 90-degree mark. Repeat for your TUL.

Shrug. Shrugs can be performed on many pieces of equipment, such as Nautilus and Hammer Strength (which have specific machines in which you sit for this exercise) or on a Universal machine's bench press station

Lateral raise (start and finish position)

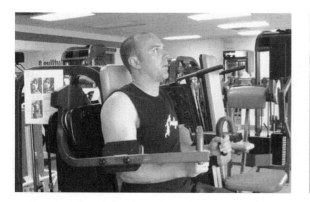
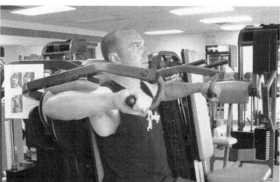

(where you would perform this exercise standing). They can also be effectively performed with dumbbells or a barbell; the former can be performed seated, while the latter should be performed standing.

When training the trapezius muscle with shrugs, make sure you're not bending your arms (as in a curl). The arms must be straight, hanging down at your sides, and only the contraction of the trapezius (which results in a shrugging motion) should be responsible for moving the resistance. Whether you're using free weights or machines, shrug slowly until your shoulders have been drawn up as high as they can possibly go. Pause briefly in the position of full muscular contraction, and then lower your shoulders until they are as low as they can go. At this point, reverse direction, and repeat the movement for your TUL.

Lower-Back Machine. Enter the lower-back machine so that the pad is on your upper back, just above the lumbar region, and your feet are on the platform. Fasten the seat belt to keep from shifting in the seat during the exercise. Place your hands either on your shoulders or in front of your abdomen. Slowly lean back until your lower-back musculature is fully contracted. Pause briefly in this position of full contraction, and then return slowly to the starting position. Repeat for your TUL.

If you are using free weights, either the dead lift or bent-over barbell row will suffice to stimulate your lower-back musculature.

Nautilus shrug (start and finish position)

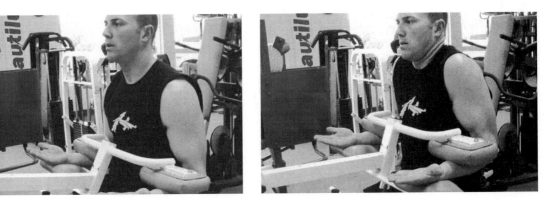

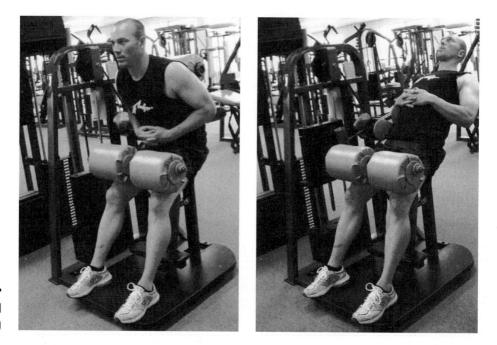

Nautilus lower back (start and finish position)

Biceps Curl. If using a machine, sit down in the biceps curl machine and place your elbows on the pads. Your elbow joint should be aligned with the center of the cam. Take hold of the handles, and slowly contract your biceps until they are fully contracted and your forearms have moved from an extended position of full stretch to a position of full contraction. Pause

Biceps curl (start and finish position)

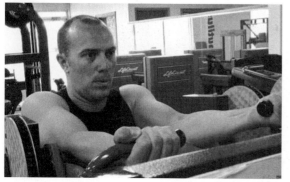
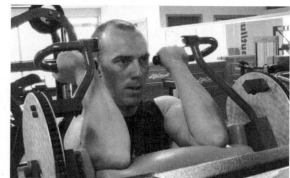

briefly in the fully contracted position, and then lower the handles back to the starting position. Repeat for your TUL.

If using free weights, take hold of a barbell with a shoulder-width grip and your palms facing forward. Stand up straight so that your knuckles are resting on your thighs. Keeping your elbows pinned in tight to your ribs, slowly curl the barbell until your hands are almost touching your shoulders. Because the effective resistance falls off at this point in a barbell curl, there is no need to pause in this position. Instead, slowly lower the barbell back to the starting position. Repeat for your TUL.

Triceps Pressdown. This exercise is to be performed on a machine that has an overhead pulley. Take hold of the handlebar with your palms facing down and your elbows pinned in to your sides. Slowly press the handlebar down until your arms are fully straight and the bar is almost touching your thighs. Pause briefly in this position of full contraction, and then slowly let the handlebar return to the starting position. Repeat for your TUL.

If you do not have access to an overhead pulley or if you are using free weights, the bench press or overhead press will provide adequate stimulation for the triceps muscles.

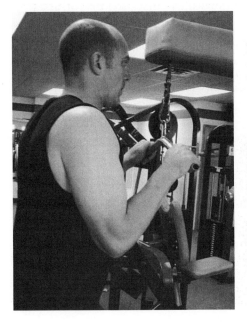 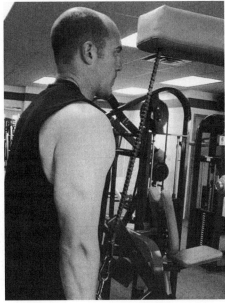

Triceps pressdown (start and finish position)

Abdominal Machine. This truly is an "optional" exercise. If you perform the pulldown exercise as previously described, there is no need to perform additional abdominal work. However, if you cannot perform the pulldown exercise, direct abdominal work isn't a bad idea. If using a machine, sit so that the pads are on your upper chest. (Some machines have handles that will be slightly above your head, in which case, take hold of these handles, making sure to keep your back on the seat pad.) Slowly contract your abdominal muscles. Don't "push" the pads with your shoulders, which will result in your torso's moving forward and downward. The range of motion for the abdominals is not great, so the distance you move will be minimal. Proceed until your abdominal muscles are fully contracted. Pause briefly in this position of full muscular contraction, and then reverse direction under control until you have returned to the starting position. Do not let the weights touch down on the stack, which would unload your abdominal muscles. Repeat for your TUL.

If you do not have access to an abdominal machine, you can perform "crunches." Simply lie down on your back on the floor. Draw your heels up as close to your buttocks as possible, and spread your knees. With your hands across your abdomen, slowly contract your abdominals until they are fully contracted. Pause briefly in this position, and then return slowly and under control to the starting position. As with the instructions for using an abdominal machine, do not let the tension come off the abdominals when you return to the starting position. Repeat for your TUL.

More on the Split Routine

I was doing the Big Three for a while, and my progress—particularly on the leg press—had slowed. Two things happened that made me reevaluate my training the whole body with the Big Three once a week.

One was that I had a trainer (Blair Wilson) who is a bright guy and is well versed in high-intensity training theory. One day, I said, "I think I'm going to change things up today, maybe do leg extensions or something," and he said, "No, you're not." I asked, "What do you mean?" He

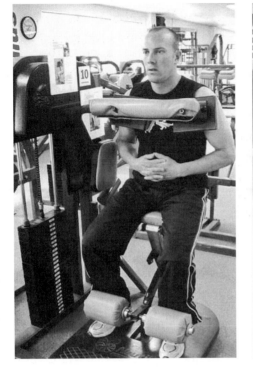
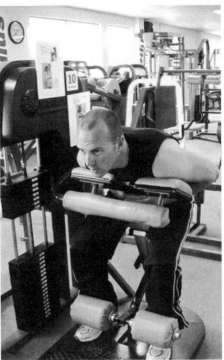

Nautilus abdominal machine (start and finish position)

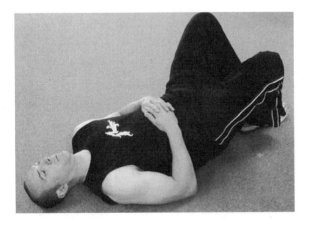
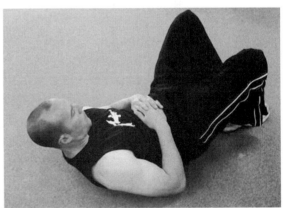

Crunch (start and finish position)

said, "Either you're going to do the leg press or you're not recovered yet." I thought, "You know, he has a point there." The first indicator of overtraining, from my perspective, is not having an inclination to train hard, and the leg press represented this huge energy output that I had to be willing and able to entertain. Moreover, my progress on that exercise had been minimal: I might have held at a certain weight and number of repetitions one week and perhaps gone up one rep the next week, and that one-rep increase might have come because of a slight loosening of my form.

The second thing that happened was that my son Riley was using Mike Mentzer's program of a three-way split routine performed once a week. Riley was sixteen years old at the time, so his hormonal levels were perfect for building muscle, and he was making great progress. I thought, "That's what I'm going to do: I'll hold off training legs for three weeks and just bite the bullet." When I returned to the leg press three weeks later, I exceeded my previous best by fifteen repetitions per leg. (I use the Nautilus duo squat leg press machine.) That just told me that the recovery period, at least for legs, is considerably longer than seven days. So, a three-way split wherein each body part gets trained once every twenty-one days was just perfect.

—John Little

When to Use the Split Routine

A split routine should be invoked as soon as the trainee witnesses a slowdown in recordable progress with the more basic, whole-body routines. If, for instance, after two workouts of the Big Five or the Big Three, there has been no progress in the amount of weight lifted or the amount of repetitions (or both), then it is time to move on to a three-way split routine. There will come a time in everyone's training career that will bring the trainee face to face with the limits of his or her genetic potential. At this stage, switching to a three-way split routine that allows for training more intensely, more briefly, and less frequently will enable the trainee to take the final step up the ladder.

Any of the aforementioned techniques can help in surmounting mechanical obstacles, allowing a trainee to reach the critical threshold necessary to stimulate continued muscular progress. This doesn't mean that these protocols result in better outcomes, nor that the goal of an increase in size and strength could not be obtained by more basic means (i.e., positive failure). Literature on the performance of negative-only exercise has revealed that the technique is effective in stimulating the production of a lean increase and strength increase, but there also is literature showing that conventional exercise methods produce increases in size and strength and that motionless (static) exercise likewise produces such increases. That said, no research has come to our attention indicating that any protocol produces results beyond the boundaries of one's genetic potential.

My Experience with the Three-Way Split Routine

With med school and residency and even my job, being fatigued and tired all the time and pushing through it is something that I'm used to doing. So, if I get in the wrong mind-set, I will train before it's time to train. Psychologically, it's easy for me to adopt the position that "The day has come: I've got to stick to the scheduled workout regardless of how I feel." To quash that inclination and keep myself in line, I have to set up a scenario that deliberately holds me back.

I'm now onto a cycle along the lines of what Mike Mentzer suggested, which calls for rotating the body in thirds once a week. I will perform two cycles of that, and then I return to a workout in which I split the body in half, working half the muscles with three exercises in one workout and the other half with three exercises the next. So, I'll do the three-way split for two cycles, followed by one cycle of the two half-body workouts, and then return to the three-way split routine again.

I've not witnessed any decompensation as a result of spreading the workouts for each bodypart out to once every twenty-one days. If anything, every muscle group has grown bigger, stronger, and fuller. At the end of one workout, when I see what my performance was, I project what the weight will be the next time that particular workout comes up in my cycle.

Since I've been doing this rotation, whenever that next workout comes up, I plug in the weight that I projected from my last workout, and every time—without fail—it's too light.

—Doug McGuff, M.D.

Max contraction

An alternate training modality that has also proved effective in overcoming sticking points and stimulating muscular growth is the Max Contraction protocol, in which a muscle is taken into its position of full contraction, and then this position is held until the contraction can no longer be sustained (typically within the same time under load as conventional full-range exercise). This protocol is ideally performed with isolation exercises.

Since the protocol is performed in the muscle's strongest point in the range of motion (the fully contracted position), the speed bump is a nonissue, and the stimulus is applied to the muscle with virtually no wear-and-tear problems. This is a significant asset, because the less wear and tear you accumulate throughout your training career, the better off you are. With a motionless protocol, you can stimulate strength and size increases that are at least equal to those obtainable with full-range training, and since muscle building is the goal, if it can occur with the least amount of wear and tear possible, this is a desirable option.

The most important quality of Max Contraction as a protocol is that it allows you to contract your muscles against a heavier load. That produces not only inroad but also the accumulated by-products of fatigue, and it does it without movement (making it safe) and without your necessarily having to concern yourself with the problem of sticking points or limitations of the equipment.

Sample Exercise Breakdown

For an effective Max Contraction workout, the trainee should select twelve exercises and create three workouts of four exercises each, to be performed on an alternating basis once every seven days. The breakdown might be as follows:

Workout 1
1. Leg extension
2. Leg curl
3. Standing calf raise
4. Abdominal crunch

Workout 2
1. Pullover
2. Lower back machine
3. Shrug
4. Arm cross

Workout 3
1. Lateral raise
2. Rear deltoid
3. Biceps curl
4. Triceps extension

The time under load for the exercises should be approximately sixty to ninety seconds (or whatever the ideal time signature is for the individual trainee), and trainees should attempt to stay within that TUL. Heavier weights can be employed to good effect if a trainer or training partner helps in lifting the load and transferring it onto the muscle group being trained. Max Contraction is an excellent tweaking stimulus in that it eliminates all momentum; no learning curve is required; and it loads the muscle thoroughly and provides ample levels of inroad, fatigue, accumulated by-products of fatigue, and stimulation for growth. Ample data in the scientific literature support the premise that a Max Contraction or constant-tension, motionless protocol produces significant strength-building effects.[5]

Compound Exercises and Max Contraction

The benefits just indicated can also be obtained with compound exercises, such as those that constitute the Big Five, but with these, you have to be careful not to lock out your limbs fully. Often the position of full contraction on a compound exercise is also the point in the range of motion of minimum movement arm. The best way to overcome this obstacle and thus impart a higher-level stimulus to your musculature is to find a fixed point in the range of motion in which you feel the force output in that particular exercise as being maximal, and then perform your set in that position. For instance, two-thirds of the way up in a leg press and just beyond the halfway point in a chest press would be good locations to perform your holds. Doing so will ensure that you are performing a legitimate maximum contraction and that your force output is the highest. The tradeoff may be that some fibers will not be producing maximum force in these positions, but it's a positive tradeoff, because you will be reducing the wear and tear associated with full-range exercise.

This is a more intense technique, so we recommend that when you implement this protocol, you perform no more than three or four exercises in a given workout—such as the leg press, pulldown, chest press, and seated row. As always, you should train no more than once a week when employing this technique, and if your training record indicates a slowdown in progress, don't be hesitant to recover further and push the frequency out to once every ten days or so.

Maintenance is regression

At no time in your training should you decide that your progress is "good enough" and elect to back off on your intensity to "maintain" your present level of size and strength. We have found that whenever this occurs, the inevitable result is a regression. We're not sure why this is, but we have witnessed this phenomenon enough to conclude that the body needs a continual challenge.

We have both had clients tell us, "I don't need to be any stronger, and I don't want to gain any more strength." If we then attempt to hold them at, say, a 200-pound pulldown and a time under load of ninety seconds (assuming this to be their capability as expressed in their previous workout), within three to four workouts, we will find them struggling to make seventy seconds with that weight. If, instead of attempting to freeze them at this level, we progress them even by a quarter of a foot-pound every workout, we have found that they will hold stable or improve slightly. Likewise, if we engage a protocol (such as the ones detailed in this chapter) that allows them to progress their weight while working around sticking points, they will continue to experience a strength progression. However, trying to hold someone's strength stable by employing the same weights and time under load simply doesn't work.

Many trainees, particularly as they grow stronger, don't like the feeling of exerting a lot of energy and are looking to pacify themselves by doing *something* but not working out "too hard." They want to work out by doing something with their muscles, but they're not keen on pushing to the level necessary to stimulate continued improvement. When this happens, we usually prescribe a little more time off between their workouts, or else we'll alter their protocol along the lines indicated in this chapter. This variation provides a psychological stimulus of doing something "new." If we change the emphasis to a protocol such as SuperSlow that emphasizes the accumulated by-products of fatigue, they feel satisfied because their muscles are still working hard but they're not lifting as heavy a load.

We recognize that some people have a pronounced fear of heavier weights, which creates an imposing psychological barrier, so we progress them over time with the different protocol. We don't change anything until roughly a year or so, and then we employ techniques and protocols on a progressive basis to keep them gaining.

USE ULTRA-INTENSITY PROTOCOLS SPARINGLY

All of the techniques and methods set forth in this chapter have to be used systematically and sparingly, because (the foregoing discussion notwithstanding) it can be all too tempting to push on to the next level— particularly for someone who is highly motivated. These methods represent a quantum leap in placing demands on the body, so overtraining can sneak up on you, and progress will grind to a halt.

Overtraining is a process, rather than an event, and it is often difficult to recognize when it's starting to happen, despite the fact that the victim has been growing progressively weaker. The best remedy for overtraining is to prevent it from happening in the first place, by deliberately mapping out ahead of time when you're going to employ these techniques and planning to use them conservatively for a short period, followed by a briefer workout program that is reduced in both volume and frequency.

For example, let's assume you begin training in September. You stay with the Big-Five workout for five months—September, October, November, December, and January. Then, starting in February, certain modifications might be made, with the full calendar year structured along the following lines:

> January—Big-Five baseline program (positive failure only)
> February—Big Five with the addition of segmented manual assistance on the leg press, chest press, and pulldown exercises
> March—Negative-only on a three-exercise program (e.g., pulldown, overhead press, leg press)
> April—Big-Five baseline program (positive failure only)
> May—Three-way split routine (with rest-pause rep after positive failure)
> June—Three-way split routine (with Max Contraction)
> July—Big Three (pulldown, chest press, leg press) taken to positive failure only
> August—Three-way split routine (with timed static contraction at the end of positive-failure sets)
> September—Three-way split routine (negative-only on each exercise)
> October—Big Three (positive failure only)
> November—Three-way split routine (with partial repetitions, performed after the sticking point in the leg press and overhead press, and performed before the sticking point in the pulldown)
> December—Three-way split routine (with segmented manual resistance on each exercise)

ENERGY CONSERVATION AND INCREASED LOAD

During periods when a trainee is employing single-axis exercises (such as a three-way split routine), caution must be taken. Not only can the body learn how to cheat to accomplish the assumed objective of making more weight go up and down, but also sometimes the mechanics of the movement make isolation impossible. For these reasons, we prefer that most exercises in a workout program be compound movements.

We've found on certain biceps machines that as the weight increases, all of a sudden a mechanical lever effect intercedes where the weight on the machine actually lifts the trainees' body out of the seat. Thus, the trainee starts using ancillary musculature just to remain stabilized in the machine and perform the movement with the heavier amount of weight. The mechanics of that exercise with that amount of force on the movement arm compels the trainee to cheat by shifting around in the apparatus. That's also true of a lot of other single-joint movements. You'll find it occurring, for instance, in the leg extension: once you get to higher levels of resistance (on a Nautilus leg extension, say, it could be anywhere from 180 to 200 pounds), it's almost impossible to keep your rear end from lifting up out of the seat.

To remedy this situation, many trainees will grip the handles on the machine really hard (which they shouldn't do as this can raise blood pressure) or seat-belt themselves into the machine, which has the consequence of producing sufficiency, because when a belt is cinched down on top of the quadriceps, this muscle group becomes compressed and cannot fully contract. In short, once a trainee ascends to more meaningful levels of resistance in these single-joint movements, it becomes almost impossible not to cheat to some degree simply because of mechanical forces.

Don't infer that you should avoid single-joint movements throughout your training career, but the core of your workout (away from Max Contraction routines) needs to be compound movements. Further, your judgment of how you're progressing needs to be based on the pieces of equipment that keep cheating to a minimum.

In conclusion, it is important to view the tweaking methods featured in this chapter not so much as *higher*-intensity techniques to employ in an effort to get the body to deliver more than it is capable of delivering, but rather as mechanisms by which to continue to progress as always, while working around the limitations of the equipment and the finite recovery capability of the human body. They are, in effect, a means by which you can raise your genetic-potential needle up from 98 percent to 100 percent.

The Genetic Factor

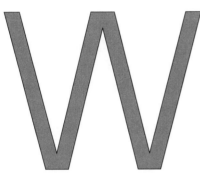

With special thanks to Ryan Hall, who researched and synthesized much of the material in this chapter.

While proper exercise can deliver exceptional results, if your desires are not firmly rooted in reality, you may well end up disappointed. Strength training is, without question, one of the most productive activities in which people can engage, yet many women avoid it for fear that they'll end up looking like Arnold Schwarzenegger, and many men who once did it quit in frustration because their bodies didn't morph into something more resembling Arnold Schwarzenegger. In the case of the women, their fears are typically unfounded, and for the men, their disappointment is normal, given that building large muscles is a rare trait in human beings. That rareness is what makes for its appeal among the masses, while the fact that this rareness is popularized in bodybuilding and fitness publications as "possible for anyone" is what makes for the fear among many women.

A LESSON FROM ECONOMICS

In the field of economics, the value of a given object is not always directly related to its importance. A lot of times, value is a function of supply relative to demand, which is how prices are typically determined. For instance, what is more valuable: diamonds or water? It is clear from the standpoint of human survival and health that water is the more valuable commodity, yet diamonds are much more expensive. The reason? Modern technology makes water abundant, so the supply relative to the demand is generally well matched. Consequently, the price is low. However, if you were stranded on a desert island where water wasn't so abundant, you would certainly opt for a bottle of water over a bag of diamonds. Similarly, extreme levels of muscularity and muscle size are rare physical qualities. They hold appeal precisely because of their rarity—and the reason for this rarity is genetics.

Three major theories formulated during the past two hundred years contributed fundamentally to the understanding of human biology and the body's "inner" world: the cell theory of German biologists Jackob Schlieden and Theodor Schwann in 1839, the theory of evolution by Charles Darwin during the 1850s, and Louis Pasteur's theory of disease in the 1860s. These contributions laid the groundwork for the most important breakthrough in the life sciences: the discovery of DNA (deoxyribonucleic acid) in 1944 by O. T. Avery. DNA forms the basis of all life. It determines the nature of every living organism on the phylogenetic scale, from its lowest single-celled entity to humans.

Within the core of DNA are genes, which "carry" the characteristics one has inherited from one's parents, who inherited them from their parents, and so on. Almost everything about you—your hair color, foot size, and even the shape and size of your muscles—is determined by genes that were transmitted by your progenitors. While anyone can fulfill his or her genetic potential for such indexes as strength and muscle size through proper training and sound nutrition, there remain limits to that potential, and these limits too are set by genetics.[1]

The ability to develop muscles beyond normal size requires the genetic structure to do so, and the naked truth is that most people do not have that genetic structure. Evolutionary biology makes certain of this because the need for that trait is relatively rare, so the process through which that sort of musculature is selected occurs infrequently, but it has not been completely eliminated.

DETERMINING FACTORS

During the late 1970s, Mike Mentzer, a bodybuilding champion and pre-med student, proposed that out of a cross section of one hundred thousand males, perhaps twenty would have the genetics to be champion bodybuilders and develop that level of muscle mass. Of those twenty, perhaps ten would even be interested in doing so, and of that ten, perhaps only one would know how to train and diet properly to give full expression to his muscular potential. This accounting would make the odds of your obtaining such a high level of development one in a hundred thousand.

While it is difficult to accurately assess an individual's genetic capacity for building bigger muscles, there are certain physical traits that an informed observer can spot. These visible characteristics, as delineated in the following sections, offer a guide to where one might be headed and indicate areas that may yield better than average potential to increase in size as a result of training.

Somatotype

While an infinite variety of body types can be encountered, authorities have concluded that three readily identifiable types recur most often. In the 1940s, American psychologist William Sheldon categorized individual bodies by analyzing the degree to which each of these three types was present. He called his system somatotyping. The three somatotypic variables are endomorphy, mesomorphy, and ectomorphy.

Endomorphy refers to the tendency toward soft, round body contours; a typical endomorph is rotund, having a round torso, a thick neck, and short, fat legs and arms. Mesomorphy refers to the tendency toward being muscular; a true mesomorph is built square and strong, with shoulders that are broad and muscular and a powerful chest and limbs, and carries little bodyfat. Ectomorphy refers to the tendency toward skinniness; an ectomorph is usually tall and always thin in the torso and limbs, with little bodyfat or muscle.

Muscle Length

Other factors can also dictate the ultimate size that one's muscles can become. Key among them is the length of the muscle. Muscle is made up of the muscle belly, which is the meat of the muscle, and the tendon on either end—which is why a muscle is called a musculotendinous unit. The greater the mass of that musculotendinous unit, the more material is available for growth. The length of a muscle is set by where its tendons anchor it to bone, so there is no means of increasing it. As a muscle's width is never going to exceed its length (because if it could, contraction would not occur), for any given muscle, the limiting factor to its volume—length × width × height—is that genetically fixed length.

Still, there is some wiggle room within the formula. An individual who may have short muscle bellies in his biceps does not necessarily possess short muscles throughout the rest of his body. The length of any specific muscle seems to be a random feature within any given person's musculature, with differences usually existing from one side of the body to the other and from one bodypart to the next. It is the extremely rare person who has uniform muscle length and/or size over the entire body.

Skeletal Formation

In assessing an individual's predisposition toward building a massive musculature, it is essential to consider skeletal formation, which is determined by the length, thickness, and structure of the body's bones. The bodily proportions normally associated with the bodybuilder's physique are broad shoulders, narrow hips, and arms and legs of medium length.

Fat Distribution

Just as people are genetically programmed to increase the size of certain muscles, they also inherit a certain number of fat, or adipose, cells. The distribution of these cells is genetically determined as well. On average, nonobese people have approximately 25 billion to 30 billion fat cells; moderately obese people have about 50 billion; and extremely obese people have as many as 240 billion. This wide range may help explain why some exceedingly overfat people find it a near impossibility to lose fat permanently.

Neuromuscular Efficiency

Neuromuscular efficiency refers to the relationship between the nervous system and the muscles. How muscles are innervated and how they are activated by the brain determine the degree of muscle power and the number of fibers required to produce a certain movement against a certain resistance. People with high levels of neuromuscular efficiency have the ability to contract a greater percentage of fibers during a maximal effort. In an all-out effort, the average person may contract 30 percent of the fibers within a specific muscle, and a few may have the capacity to activate as many as 40 percent, while even fewer can manage 50 percent. The ability to contract a high percentage of fibers increases contractile capacity and thus enables more intense exertion. In matters of endurance, this endowment is a disadvantage, but it is a definite advantage for stimulating muscle growth, sprinting, and single-attempt efforts.

Muscle-Fiber Density

Muscle-fiber density is a measure of the number of individual muscle fibers per cubic centimeter. The more fibers you have per cubic centimeter, the more you have available to be stimulated to hypertrophy. Since you cannot stimulate growth in fibers that do not exist, the more fibers you have, the greater will be the mass potential of any given muscle.

Muscle Shape and Size Potential

Muscles come in two distinctly different shapes, and it is the manner in which fibers are arranged within a muscle that determines if that particular muscle has the potential to increase its size. These two classic fiber shapes are fusiform and pennate.

A fusiform muscle is shaped like a football. An example is the biceps muscle of the upper arm. Because of its shape, this muscle has considerable ability to increase its volume.

In pennate muscles, the fibers are arranged more like the fronds of a feather. This arrangement creates a pulling angle that gives them a hefty force advantage over their fusiform counterparts. However, pennate fibers are layered such that they're only a few fibers thick, as opposed to being layered around and around like a jelly roll, as fusiform fibers are. These muscles are arranged this way because they're located in small spaces; if they were fusiformed, every increase in power output would result in a decrease in the muscle's functional ability, owing to an increase in the cross-sectional area of the muscle.

An example of a pennate muscle is the interosseous muscle between the bones of the hand. This muscle comes into play whenever gripping is required. If it had the mass potential of a fusiform muscle, you would soon develop a hand shaped like a balloon, and its functional ability in gripping would be lost. Similarly, the soleus, which is sandwiched on the side of your calf, has to fit between your gastrocnemius and the posterior edge of your tibia. If this muscle were to enlarge significantly, it would displace your gastrocnemius in a posterior direction such that its pulling angle would be compromised, and it would lose strength. From this description, it should be obvious that certain muscles are arranged in this pennate fashion in order to *avoid* significant increases in volume. The natural consequence is that some muscles will never increase in size in any meaningful way, owing to their shape. It isn't in the genetic cards.

Myostatin

The vast majority of the population, as has been documented, do not bear the requisite physical characteristics to develop supranormal-size muscles, and for good biologic reason. From our evolutionary ancestors' standpoint, the ability to easily develop large muscles would be a principal disadvantage to surviving in an environment of food scarcity such as existed back then. Muscle is metabolically active tissue, and sustaining and supporting even a normal-size musculature is a trial when energy is scarce, so it would be well-nigh out of the question for people with supranormal levels of this tissue, because of its high caloric demands.

Reluctant as a trainee may be to accept it, there is a distinct evolutionary disincentive for having too much muscle—and a related need for an internal mechanism that constrains how large the muscles can become. Nature has answered that need by providing myostatin.

A specific gene, named growth and differentiation factor 8 (GDF-8), produces this protein, the function of which is to stop muscle stem cells or satellite cells from becoming larger. GDF-8 in effect controls the borders on how large muscles can become. Most people have a generous expression of this GDF-8 gene and therefore have a considerable amount of myostatin circulating through their bodies, which imposes a modest limit on how much muscle mass their bodies will produce.

Myostatin was first noted in Belgian cattle. Although there is not much open plain in Belgium, the country's cattle breeders nevertheless were able to produce a type of bull with up to 30 percent more muscle mass than the average bovine. It was evidently through selective breeding over time that they subsequently created a Herculean strain of bull now known as the Belgian blue, the unique feature of which is that it carries two to three times more muscle mass than standard beef cattle. (In the United States, a similar process of selective breeding has resulted in a breed of cattle called the Piedmontese.)

Knowing that more beef on the hoof equates to more meat yield, and hence more money to be made per head of cattle, researchers began to look into why the Belgian blue was so freakishly large. To their surprise, they discovered that this strain of cattle was lacking a gene (GDF-8) that encoded for the myostatin protein, and they believed that this difference was why these cattle had become so muscular.

Researchers Se-Jin Lee and Alexandra McPherron, from Johns Hopkins University, tested that theory by subjecting littermate mice (essentially twin mice) to a process that resulted in postnatal deletion of the GDF-8 gene. What they observed was that the mice became phenomenally over-muscled. This research confirmed that the lack of expression of GDF-8 was the cause of the excess musculature.[2]

The data from these researchers stimulated considerable interest within the scientific community and spurred additional research involving similar genetic knockouts in other animals—with identical results. Once scientists realized that they could knock out this gene and produce a predictable result, they knew they had successfully identified the gene (and its expressed protein) responsible for the unprecedented muscle-building effect. Interest in this research quickly spread to the human realm when it became apparent that muscle-wasting conditions such as muscular dystrophy, AIDS, starvation, and cancer could all benefit from a manipulation of this gene in humans.

In this endeavor, the scientists wanted to determine if there was a way to achieve the muscle-building effect without the harshness of deleting the gene in question. A lot of genes encode for multiple proteins or signals, and if you knock out an entire gene, you might produce some negative effects in the process of acquiring the beneficial effect. Within this context, rather than trying to develop a drug that would knock the gene out, researchers began to turn their attention to finding a means by which to bind up the gene's product protein so as to inhibit its expression. The first compound they investigated was follistatin, which is typically employed to treat hormonal disorders of the hypothalamic pituitary axis.

In 1997, they were pleased to discover that follistatin could in fact bind certain hormones over their receptor surface and thus prevent their expression. The best way to envision this process is to think of myostatin as a key, with follistatin as an agent that covers up the ridges of the key so that it no longer fits its receptor keyhole. This as opposed to another agent that might cover the myostatin key but not cover the key ridges—it might cover the handle of the key instead. Follistatin was found to work well in this regard, effectively binding the myostatin and inhibiting its function. Researchers were thus able to produce a double-muscling effect by covering up the protein at its interface with the receptor, instead of knocking out the gene in toto.

A damper on their success was the problem that the effect was not isolated: while follistatin did bind the protein, it also bound other hormones. So, back to the drawing board they went to work on developing a more specific, monoclonal type of antibody. They needed something that would be specific to the myostatin protein in blocking its functioning within the body. This attempt was successful and resulted in patents for compounds by a company called Metamorphix, an enterprise started up with venture capital money, and the principals of which were researchers Lee and McPherron. Metamorphix held the patents on the rights to this product for use in animal fields, such as animal husbandry, while the rights to the human version of the drug were sold to Wyeth Pharmaceuticals.

To make the leap from animal research to human research, it was important that a human example of a spontaneous myostatin deletion be discovered. The researchers needed to be able to demonstrate that myostatin deletion occurred naturally (albeit rarely) in humans; otherwise, approval from the Human Research Advisory Committee would be withheld, preventing research from being conducted with humans. So, in the ensuing years, from 1998 through 2004, an incredible manhunt was under way to find human examples of myostatin deletion.

McPherron and Lee began taking blood samples from bodybuilders, and author Doug McGuff was sent blood collection kits to try to obtain samples from individuals who he thought would be likely candidates. This approach came up empty all around. The reason had nothing to do with fear of needles; it was all about money. Obtaining a blood sample required the subject's informed consent, which was predicated on a full understanding of what the researchers were trying to establish with that sample—that extreme, impressive muscularity is a gift of genetics and not the result of a specific training, drug, or supplement protocol. It quickly became evident that a lot of the people who had this gift bestowed on them by nature are able to use it not just for winning athletic competitions and bodybuilding contests but also for lucrative endorsements of a host of products, the most prominent being their own training programs or food supplements. To establish in the public eye that they in fact had this myostatin deletion would extremely compromise their marketability.

While researchers were coming up short with professional athletes, a breakthrough occurred when, in the June 24, 2004, edition of the *New England Journal of Medicine*, it was announced that a myostatin mutation had been discovered in a toddler in Germany.[3] This announcement opened the floodgates for scientists to proceed with human testing, and a human version was developed. Named Myo-O29, it underwent phase one trials but has rather suspiciously dropped from the radar since then.

While this flurry of research was going on, other animal species were showing up that, through selective breeding, were likewise developing the myostatin deletion. In the world of dog racing, to cite a prime example, this development has become a formidable controversy. A lot of the best racing dogs are whippets, and time and again, the whippets that were winning the most races appeared to be extremely muscular. When this circumstance came to the attention of researchers, they started testing these animals and discovered that, through selective breeding, these types of whippets (which are now called bully whippets) have the myostatin deletion.[4] If you look in your search engine for "Wendy the Muscular Whippet," you will be flabbergasted at how muscular a normally skinny little whippet can be.

A lack of myostatin can manifest not only in inordinate levels of muscle size but also in lower levels of bodyfat. The bonus is that both of these effects seem to be produced concurrently, making the subject highly defined in appearance—or "ripped," as the bodybuilders like to say.[5]

To reiterate, the extremely muscular look that so many women fear they might acquire if they strength-train, and that so many men crave, would seem to be under the exclusive control of one's level of myostatin. Those who have bigger muscles and those with the most potential to develop tremendous muscle mass are, like it or not, those who have slipped through the evolutionary cracks. After something that could produce a rapid increase in muscle tissue, which could, in turn, chew up enough calories to rapidly reduce bodyfat levels (our reserve tank in times of famine) would not have much survival value.

In addition to myostatin, there are other genetic determinants of what your response to training might be and your potential muscle size, as well as how specific alterations in a training protocol can be custom tailored to allow these genetic traits full expression. These genetic factors include ciliary neurotrophic factor (CNTF), interleukin-15, alpha-actinin-3, myosin light chain kinase, and angiotensin converting enzyme.[6]

Ciliary Neurotrophic Factor (CNTF)

Ciliary neurotrophic factor is a chemical that promotes survival of motor units. CNTF declines with age, but an injection of this chemical into aged lab animals has been shown to significantly increase their strength and muscle mass. The relative presence or absence of CNTF can also affect potential muscle size.

Interleukin-15

The gene combinations of interleukin-15 are closely associated with positive responses to resistance exercise. Interleukin-15 is expressed by three different gene possibilities (known as "genotypes"): Type AA, Type CA, and Type CC. In terms of response in muscle size after exposure to resistance exercise, the AA genotype of interleukin-15 produces a much greater increase than the CC genotype, which has minimal to no effect in that area, while the CA genotype produces an intermediate or modest response. However, in regard to muscle strength in response to strength training, the opposite extremes pertain: the AA genotype produces the least strength increase (but the most mass increase), while the CC genotype produces the greatest strength increase (even though it produces the least mass increase). The CA genotype again produces a more modest or intermediate response. Add it all up, and the interleukin-15 genotype can factor in determining someone's size and strength responses to resistance exercise.

Alpha-Actinin-3

Alpha-actinin-3 is a component of the actin filament in the myofibril of fast-twitch skeletal muscle. Across the general population, roughly 18 percent of people lack this protein entirely. Narrowing the focus, though, to only athletes presents an entirely different composition: no world-championship sprinters to date have been shown to lack alpha-actinin-3, while one-third of all champion endurance athletes lack it.[7] It certainly appears that if you're going to be a power- or speed-based athlete, it would behoove your genome to be in possession of alpha-actinin-3. As for its role in response to strength training, some preliminary studies indicate that people who lack alpha-actinin-3 tend to benefit more from strength training than those who possess it. A caveat is that some of these studies have come under criticism because the protocols that were used to test that hypothesis were relatively high in volume and consequently relatively low in intensity. It is postulated that if a lower-volume/higher-intensity training program had been employed, subjects with alpha-actinin-3 would have fared better.

Myosin Light Chain Kinase

Myosin light chain kinase is an enzyme that involves the coupling of the myosin and actin filaments on the myosin light chain. The more of this protein you have, the more cross-bridges you can develop, and therefore the more strength you can express. The flip side is that the higher your expression of myosin light chain kinase, the greater is your degree of inroad with exertion, the more muscle damage you develop with exertion, and the longer the recovery interval you will require between workouts. So, if you happen to have high levels of myosin light chain kinase, you will be stronger, but you will also inroad your muscles much more deeply and therefore will have to train far less frequently to maximize your results.

Arthur Jones, the man who invented Nautilus exercise equipment and spent millions of dollars and thousands of hours conducting strength tests of various muscle groups, once spoke at West Point Military Academy. In his remarks to the cadets, he mentioned that one of the subjects he tested for strength output had started out at a markedly high level of strength, but after just a few repetitions, his strength dropped down to nearly zero. Jones assumed that the subject was not putting forth enough effort—that he wasn't trying—and summarily sent him on his way. Many years of research later, Jones realized to his dismay that he had precipitously dismissed potentially the strongest power lifter he had ever seen—and that the subject's prowess might have been directly attributable to his level of myosin light chain kinase expression.

Angiotensin Converting Enzyme

Angiotensin converting enzyme has much to do in determining vascular tone. With respect to the gene responsible, you have either an insertion gene (an "i" gene) or a deletion gene (a "d" gene). Individuals who have two copies of the insertion gene (an "ii" gene) of the angiotensin converting enzyme tend to have high levels of slow-twitch fibers and to be especially endurance oriented, while those who have a dual deletion (a "dd") have fibers that are predominantly fast twitch and therefore tend to be especially powerful and "sprint" oriented. People who have an insertion/deletion component ("i/d") typically fall somewhere in the middle. The "ii" version of this enzyme is inhibitory: it blunts the response to strength training. People with the "ii" version likely respond better to higher repetitions, longer TULs, and even multiple sets, whereas those who possess the dual deletion seem to be able to get stronger on almost any training protocol.

High-Intensity Responders

In practical terms, the genetic research discloses that with a training protocol that is especially high in intensity and low in volume, the type of trainee that is going to respond best is someone who has the alpha-actinin-3 component. By extension, this person will be more of a sprinter than a distance runner. The prime responder will also probably possess the myosin light chain kinase enzyme, which would have been inherited from both parents.

This trainee is going to experience greater strength increases from resistance exercise but will also have increased levels of muscle damage and inroad, requiring a longer recovery interval between workouts.

Moreover, this person is going to have the angiotensin converting enzyme dual deletion, along with a relatively higher percentage of fast-twitch fibers, and consequently will respond better in terms of strength to lower reps and lower sets.

Modest Intensity Responders

The trainee who is lacking alpha-actinin-3. This trainee also has lower levels of myosin light chain kinase and has the "ii" version of the angiotensin converting enzyme. A trainee who combines these three factors will be further along the continuum of responding better to a slightly lower level of intensity, which allows for a slightly higher level of volume. Still, ideals aside, there's no evidence that you can't have various combinations of these three elements that might put you anywhere along that spectrum.

The conclusion to be drawn, based on the evidence, is that genetic markers will hold sway over how good your response to proper exercise is going to be, as well as to what training protocols you will respond best. At present, the best way to measure an individual's levels of these genetic components is through muscle biopsies, which can be an impractical undertaking. Then too, most muscle biopsies are taken out of the vastus lateralis in the quadriceps muscle group, but there's nothing to say that the expression of those particular genes is going to be homogeneous throughout every muscle group in the body. For all we know, you might have a completely different combination of these genes in your pectoralis muscles.

The good news on this front is that you don't really have to know what your particular expressions of these individual genetic factors are in order to optimize your response to training. What is important is that you know they exist and that you diligently keep records of your workouts so that you can measure your progress and identify what protocols yield either a reduction or an improvement in your performance. Armed with this knowledge, you can make the necessary fine-tuning adjustments on your own so that you get the most out of every workout you perform. As long as you are getting stronger and the strength increases are not coming at the expense of your form on the exercises, you can rest assured that you are training with the correct (or optimal) intensity, volume, and frequency for your genotype.

EPIGENETICS

Yes, your genetic endowment can be either a boon or a drawback to your response to training, but this doesn't mean that unless you were dealt a full hand of genetic cards, training will bring no appreciable payoff. Regardless of the luck of the genetic draw, you can improve the effects of exercise on your body (albeit modestly) with what you do and with the choices you make. This startling discovery falls under the heading of epigenetics.

Although epigenetics is considered something of a new field in molecular biology, its origins date back to the turn of the twentieth century. Current discussions of epigenetics reference the Greek prefix *epi-*, which means "on top of" or "above." Prior to the introduction of this science, genetics was believed to operate strictly based on the sequencing of the base pairs of DNA, which encode for specific proteins that are expressed by certain genes within the body. It was assumed that any changes that could occur came about as a result of changes in the actual DNA sequencing and that this change was accomplished only through spontaneous mutation or by scientists deliberately manipulating a certain gene (such as knocking out the myostatin gene). Now, however, it has been shown that other modifications can occur to the DNA that *don't* involve changes in the DNA sequence. And these modifications work on significantly affecting how one's DNA is expressed.

Most epigenetic changes involve chemical bonds to DNA. Examples are methylation, which is the attachment of a methyl group; acetylation, the attachment of an acetyl group; phosophorylation, the attachment of a phosphoryl group; and chromatin remodeling. Chromatin remodeling is particularly worthy of note in that it produces a complex of proteins on top of the DNA that will determine the shape of the DNA inside of the nucleus. Certain types of chromatin may cause the DNA to become more tightly

THEORETICAL FUNDAMENTALS OF HIGH-INTENSITY TRAINING

The most time-efficient and productive exercise program is one based upon the principles of high-intensity training. Productive exercise must be of a threshold level of intensity (as any level below this threshold will not stimulate maximal results). As a result, high-intensity exercise sessions will be comparatively brief and infrequently performed (as opposed to conventional exercise programs).

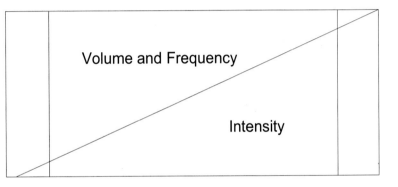

The degree to which you've been weakened, and the amount of time it took to do so (approximately two minutes), represents a threat that from the body's perspective must be addressed. The positive adaptive response to effective resistance training is the building of bigger, stronger muscles so that there will be more strength left over the next time such a stimulus is encountered. As you repeat the process, you will increase the resistance that your muscles will be made to contract against to produce a similar response each time, but doing so is metabolically expensive. As this diagram illustrates, by performing more intense exercise you must reduce the volume and frequency of that exercise, and vice versa.

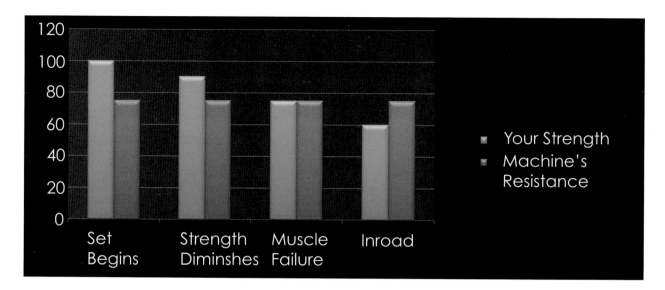

To get the best results from your high-intensity session, the authors subscribe to the **Inroad Theory of Exercise.** Inroad is *the momentary weakening of a muscle.* The graph above illustrates what happens to your strength as you perform a set of exercise. Time is indicated along the bottom (the x-axis) and units of force are represented along the side (the y-axis). The red bars represent the exercise machine's resistance (weight) holding steady at 75 units. Each set of blue and red bars represents the progression of the set and the diminishing strength of the muscles you are exercising. Here's how the phenomenon of inroading is achieved:

Stage 1: Set begins. At the beginning of the set, you are fresh with 100 units of strength (represented by the blue bar). For inroad to occur, the resistance must be meaningful, i.e., 75–80 percent of your existing strength level. If the resistance selected is too light, the muscle will recover at a faster rate than it fatigues, with the result that no inroad will occur. Using a slow, controlled speed of contraction and extension, move the weight for 6–10 seconds during the lifting (or positive) phase, and 6–10 seconds during the lowering (or negative) phase.

Stage 2: Strength diminishes. With each passing second of exercise your initial strength level diminishes, and your level of fatigue increases. Your respiration increases, and you begin to feel the burning sensation of lactic acid in your muscles. You've now lost some degree of your initial 100 units of strength (the blue bar is slowly going down), but you are still stronger than the 75 units of resistance on the machine.

Stage 3: Muscles fail. Your muscles are now so weakened that it may take you 15, 20, or even 30 seconds to complete the lifting portion of the repetition, and it is getting very difficult to control the lowering portion of the repetition. Your strength and the resistance are at virtually the same level, but your strength continues to drop until it's just below the resistance. This is where inroading begins.

Stage 4: Inroad. You attempt to move the resistance but fail to do so. You continue to do this for 10 seconds as your strength dips well below the resistance level of the machine. At the end of the countdown you unload from the machine. By the time the set is finished, your strength has been reduced to approximately 60 units, and you've inroaded your muscles by 40 percent.

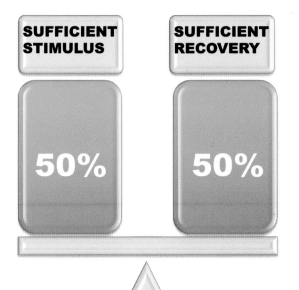

SUFFICIENT STIMULUS 50%

SUFFICIENT RECOVERY 50%

Inroading consumes resources that must be replenished. If you bring the inroading stimulus back to your muscles before your body has completed the response, it will either interfere with the response or prevent it from occurring. Providing a sufficient stimulus is only 50 percent of the process, sufficient recovery time makes up the other 50 percent. This is why you should not perform more than one workout per week.

When inroading is successfully achieved from exercise, not only is muscle growth promoted, but some secondary events take place as well:

Cardio-respiratory stimulation: Your cardio-respiratory system serves the mechanical functioning of the muscles. The higher the intensity of the muscular work, the higher the quality of the cardiovascular and respiratory stimulus will be.

Metabolic stimulation: During inroading, metabolic wastes (mostly lactic acid) accumulate faster than they can be eliminated. This creates an environment where growth factors are released and the first stages of muscle growth are stimulated.

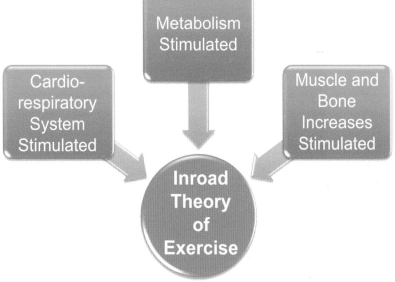

Metabolism Stimulated

Cardio-respiratory System Stimulated

Muscle and Bone Increases Stimulated

Inroad Theory of Exercise

Muscle and bone increases: As you get stronger, heavier weights are necessary to challenge you enough for inroading to occur. Exposure to heavier weights causes microscopic cellular damage that initiates the muscular adaptation and is viewed as essential for stimulating increases in bone mineral density. The illustrations on the pages that follow will look at the muscles targeted in each of the "Big-Five" exercises discussed.

Seated Row

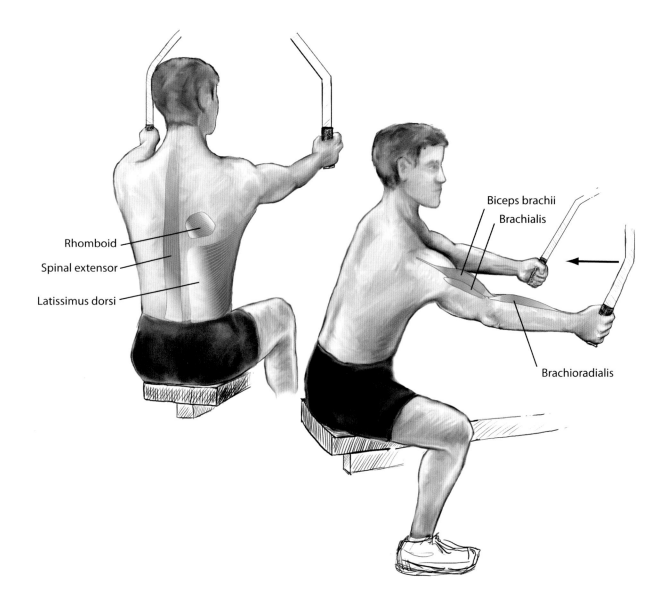

Rhomboid

Spinal extensor

Latissimus dorsi

Biceps brachii

Brachialis

Brachioradialis

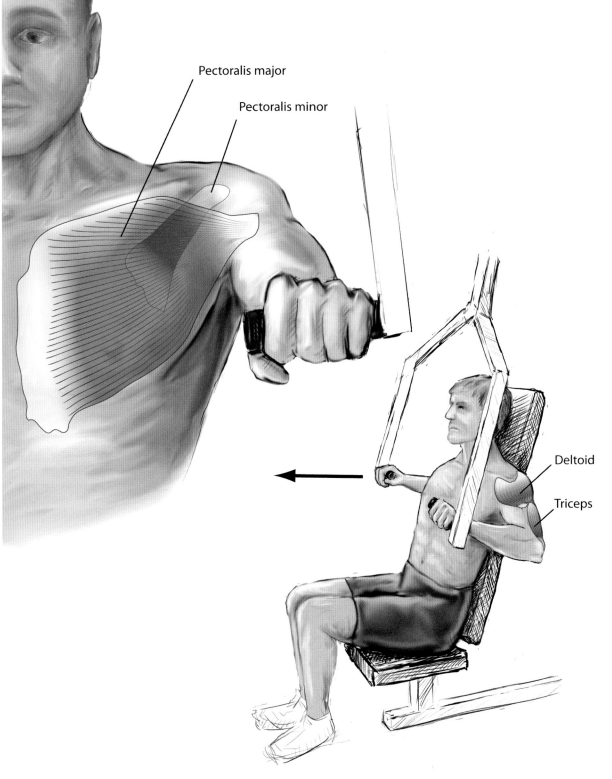

Chest Press

Pectoralis major

Pectoralis minor

Deltoid

Triceps

Pulldown

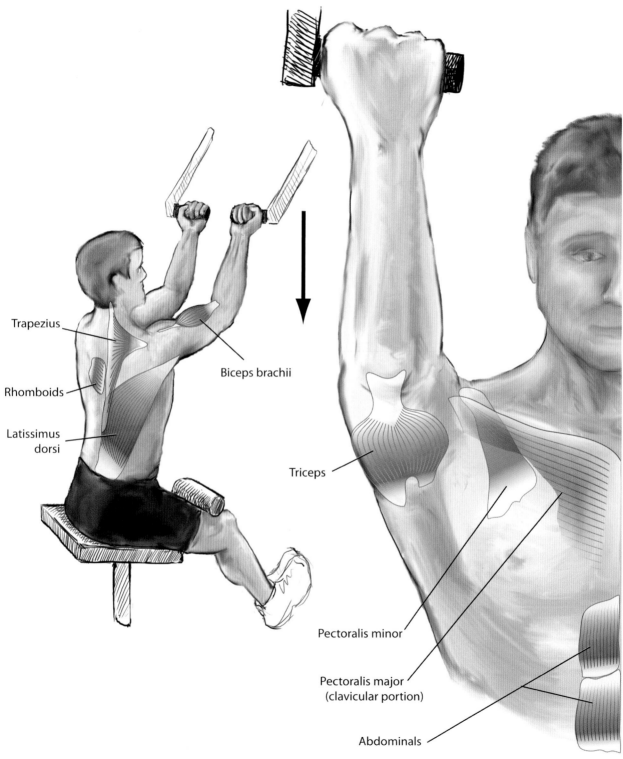

Trapezius

Rhomboids

Latissimus dorsi

Biceps brachii

Triceps

Pectoralis minor

Pectoralis major (clavicular portion)

Abdominals

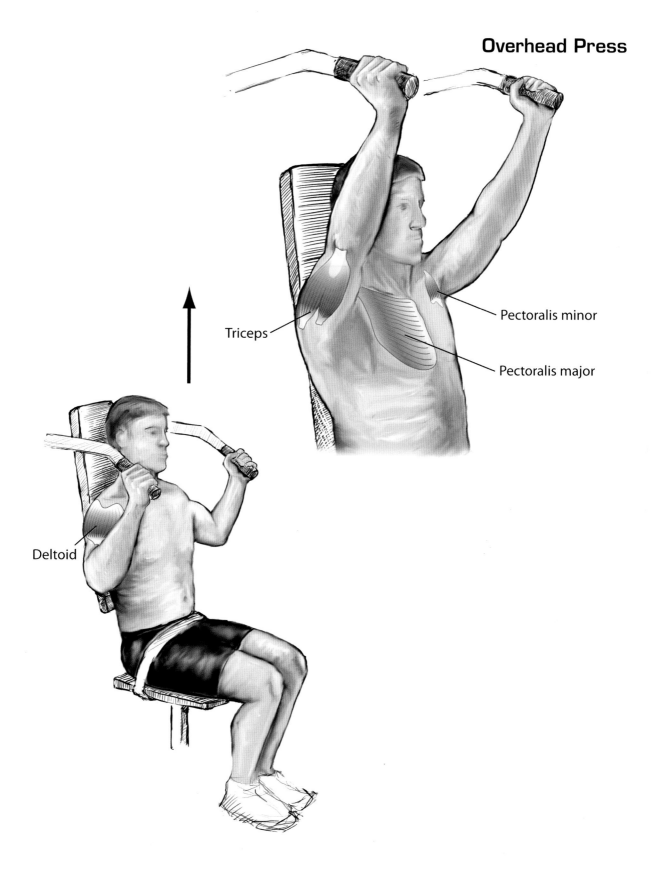

Overhead Press

Pectoralis minor

Pectoralis major

Triceps

Deltoid

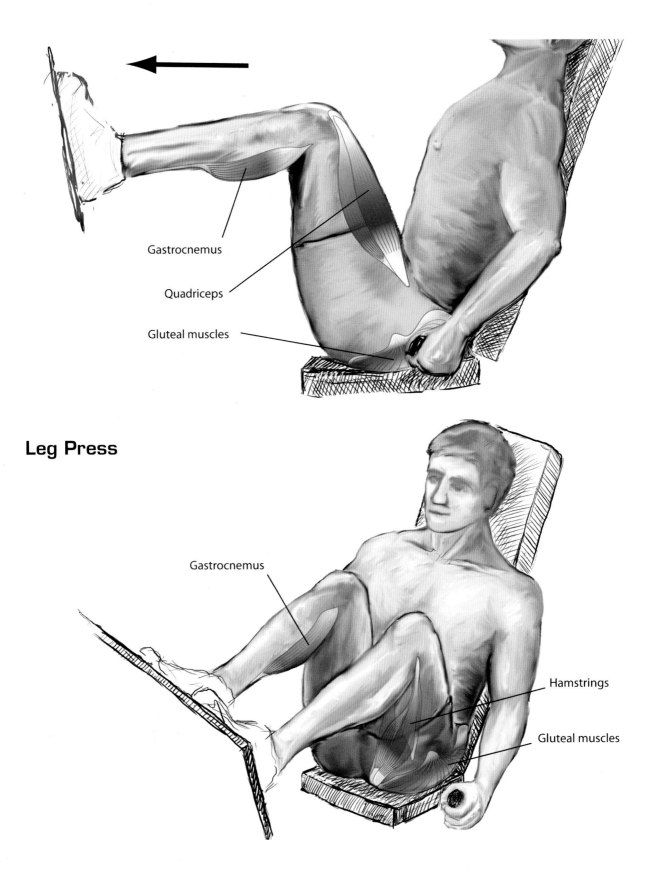

Gastrocnemus

Quadriceps

Gluteal muscles

Leg Press

Gastrocnemus

Hamstrings

Gluteal muscles

packed; when that happens, genes in these areas tend to not be expressed. Epigenetic changes can have effects on this chromatin and on how tightly packed the DNA is and, thus, can determine whether that particular gene will be expressed or ignored.

What's intriguing about these various little modifications is that they occur *on* the DNA molecule, and they occur by means of *environmental* influences. So far, the majority of epigenetic research has been done on rodents. For instance, in certain rats, the act of licking and grooming performed by the mother has been documented to create epigenetic changes on the groomed rat's genome that select either calm behavior or neurotic, anxious behavior.

THE POWER OF ENVIRONMENTAL INFLUENCE

Whereas it was once held that only changes in the DNA backbone could be passed on to offspring, scientists are now seeing that these epigenetic changes also can be passed on, for as long as four generations after the factor of influence. Two known triggers of these changes are behavioral and dietary influences. In one example, a certain strain of rat that was bred to be obese was fed a special diet containing high levels of folate, which donates methyl groups to certain genes that control metabolism and obesity. This course changed what should have been an obese rat into a lean one. The genetic change was then passed on through the rat's offspring for two to four generations.

Another example that has been noted to cause epigenetic changes in regard to obesity—although this time negative changes—is the ingestion of certain toxic compounds. Among these toxins are polyphenols, which are used in recyclable plastics and have been linked to epigenetic changes that *cause* obesity. Polyphenols are present in all sorts of plastics that are used for packaging, such as for bottled water and microwave dinners, and even in sandwich bags. There is speculation that these chemicals are among a constellation of contributors to the wave of obesity that is seen in the developed countries but that is not seen in the underdeveloped regions.

The science of epigenetics has revealed myriad environmental influences that can make such changes to human DNA and that have the power to produce consequences both for the individual and for that person's offspring. These influences vary considerably, from simple acts such as grooming to more complex variables such as diet and exercise, and are all within people's conscious control.

If you envision an immensely long strand of DNA, these epigenetic changes are like "on" and "off" switches; they either turn on or turn off a given gene. All sorts of genes when turned on inappropriately can result in disease but when not turned on, or when turned on appropriately, do not result in disease. These "switches" (actually, a long switch array) are of utmost importance to our species' health and longevity. They communicate to your DNA molecule a type of code that says in effect, "If this, then that" and "If that, then this," allowing you to turn on and turn off genes that express for health or other factors, depending on what you do.

These choices that you make are dynamic and relatively random, in that they're not linear; so, the effect is not always proportional to the cause—and sometimes is widely disproportional. While you never can predict the magnitude of the effect, you can surely predict that the lifestyle choices you make are going to directly influence the expression of your DNA and your health. This is where exercise looms large and may well have more of an influence than is currently understood. While we have made the argument in this chapter that a person's genetic potential for building muscle is pretty much fixed, the science of epigenetics points to the fact that people's choices regarding exercise and lifestyle may produce long-term positive effects on their health and on their genomes.

In the area of lifestyle choices, there is some evidence that certain epigenetic changes can occur just by virtue of a person's being in the presence of others. For instance, if you perform proper strength training and become stronger, it doesn't just mean that any children you should have in the future may carry those benefits; it also means that any previously born offspring may benefit as well, assuming they share your environment. The same applies to negative factors: some studies have indicated that a person's risk for obesity can increase by as much as 57 percent if the person habitually associates with people who are obese. One such study appeared in the July 26, 2007, *New England Journal of Medicine*.[8] So, it's not just that you pass such changes on through the act of procreation; you can also pass them on environmentally.[9]

It turns out that Mom was right all along: a person's peer group is enormously influential. If epigenetics is as powerful a component for humans as it appears to be from studies on other animals, it could have broad implications for all manner of things, including the type of exercise advocated in this book. More important, it offers hope for someone with a genetic disposition to not gain a lot of muscle mass or to become obese. There is now compelling evidence that epigenetic changes can make a difference, that people can actually change how their DNA expresses itself through environmental triggers. Perhaps the most hopeful nugget that we can present from this book's perspective is that the intelligent application of proper exercise can produce beneficial changes at a molecular level that will mean a difference for you and everyone around you, especially your offspring. It is empowering to know that you can be making a change for the better that is adaptive—and that is adaptive in a way that you get to pass on to others.

It used to be thought that human beings' ability to adapt, as well as whether certain genes would get passed on into the future, was determined by the DNA inherited at birth—and that was that. The philosophy underlying this concept was obviously deterministic, and it has never quite fit empirically. You've got to wonder why the science doesn't fit the philosophy, when the philosophy appears to be so self-evident as to what does and does not work. Upon further review, what makes more sense is to complement the determinism with a measure of free will and command over one's own destiny—and as it happens, biology backs up that revision. Within this framework, we want you to understand that by choosing the program of exercise that we offer, you are making fundamental changes that affect the "fitness of our species," so to speak.

Granted, epigenetics is still a science in its infancy, but certain things seem clear already. Chiefly, improvement through the types of steps we're endorsing in this book can have meaningful effects, tying in both the mind and the body and impacting certain psychosomatic conditions. While it's important to understand what your limitations are and not to become frustrated by them, it's also important to understand that environmental and volitional influences on how we behave can have distinct consequences corporeally. Everything about your environment in some way determines how your DNA is going to be expressed, because, as previously discussed, not only is DNA self-replicating, but also it has an interest in passing itself into the future. Consequently, it also makes sense that having some plasticity in this molecule would offer an adaptive advantage, better ensuring that the "rental car" of the body carries it forward into the future.

The Science of Fat Loss

F at is an amazing tissue. It has ensured the survival of our species through two ice ages and never-ending drought and famine. A mere pound of fat stores an astounding 3,500 calories for delayed use at any time in the future. Because it is dormant tissue, there is almost no metabolic cost for keeping it on the body. As members of the human species, we all owe our existence to fat. Even more amazing than fat's capabilities are the number of misconceptions surrounding this specialized body tissue.

FAT STORAGE

Probably the biggest misconception regarding fat is the idea that it is unhealthful. Actually, fat is probably the main reason we are even here at all. Throughout human history, the ready availability of food was the exception rather than the rule. The ability to eat when food was available and to store excess caloric energy for future use allowed people to survive when food was not at hand. Fat storage is the sign of good health, as it signals that metabolic resources are abundant and the organism is thriving. While an extreme overabundance of bodyfat places stresses on the body and can impair health, the degree of leanness (lack of bodyfat) that is currently in vogue is probably just as detrimental. Nevertheless, unhealthful levels of bodyfat have been increasing every decade. To put it bluntly, an adaptation that has allowed human beings to survive through history has now become a potential killer.

Leptin

Just as the human body has the GDF-8 gene, which encodes for myostatin, thus placing a limit on how much muscle mass a person may carry (as discussed in the previous chapter), it likewise has a genetic set point for how much bodyfat a particular individual may carry. Known as the "ob gene," it produces the protein leptin, which is a strong suppressor of appetite and food intake. As one's bodyfat level rises, more leptin is produced, causing appetite to decline, so that bodyfat levels stabilize. By the same token, if one's bodyfat level falls, leptin production declines, and appetite is disinhibited. So, it seems that we inherit a bodyfat set point that is most efficient for our environment, just as our ancestors inherited one for theirs.

The Sedentary Life?

Ask almost anyone why obesity is on the rise, and you will get a predictable answer. The common supposition is that the laborsaving technologies of modern life have made us more sedentary and that we are much less physically active than our ancestors. That is, because physical activity burns calories, and people today are less physically active than earlier populations, we are unable to burn off the calories as once was the norm. This argument seems logical, but it is incorrect on two fronts.

First, physical activity burns far fewer calories than is commonly thought. This point is further discussed later in the chapter. Suffice it to say that to survive, people must be able to use their energy efficiently lest they starve to death in the process of hunting and gathering food. Second, our ancestors were not as physically active as we romantically like to think they were. The work of anthropologists who observe primitive peoples in various regions of the globe shows a primitive hunter-gatherer lifestyle to be much less physically active than that of most of the modern world. In Australia, aborigines alternate between modernity and traditional aboriginal life, and in their more primitive mode, they are noted to be much less active. So, despite popular opinion, it does not appear that increased activity is the solution to today's obesity crisis.

The real source of modern obesity is food abundance. If we were to give you a jumbo industrial role of toilet paper and allow you to hold it while we unwind it, you would end up with a very long strand of toilet paper. If we tore off the last square, leaving you with the rest, your length of toilet paper would represent the period of human history during which starvation was a real day-to-day threat. The single square remaining would represent the period of history during which the threat of starvation had been for the most part addressed. (Obviously, there are parts of the world still suffering from food shortages.) Not since the end of the Great Depression and World War II has starvation been a real possibility in the industrialized world. For about 150,000 generations, efficient fat storage was essential for survival, but only three to four generations have seen efficient fat storage lead to obesity.

The problem is not that people today are inactive; the problem is that calories are so readily available to be consumed. Diners judge the value of their meals by the size of the portions they are given, and when people go out to eat, they want to leave feeling *full*. On this point, studies have shown that there is a difference of roughly 1,000 calories between feeling satisfied and feeling full. Moving on, there is a difference of 2,000 to 3,000 calories between feeling full and feeling stuffed. If you go out to an all-you-can-eat buffet and leave feeling stuffed, you may have consumed as many as 4,000 unneeded calories.

When this happens, people typically go out for a run the next day to "burn off those calories," but according to the calorie calculator published on the *Runner's World* website (runnersworld.com/cda/caloriecalculator), to burn off that many calories would require running continuously for almost twenty-nine miles for a 185-pound man and running almost forty-four miles for a 120-pound woman. The problem, then, is not burning too few calories; it's putting too many calories down the throat.

The Fitness Industry Lies: Exercise Doesn't Burn That Many Calories

You go to a health club and climb onto a stair stepper or treadmill, and the machine electronically prompts you to punch in numbers for your weight, select your speed or program, and begin your workout. As you plod along on the apparatus, you are motivated to keep going by an ever-increasing number on the screen that tracks the calories you have burned. After roughly one hour of this activity, the machine blinks up at you, telling you that you have burned 300 calories, and you are left with a feeling of accomplishment. Now, as you wipe the sweat from your brow and catch your breath, let us ask you a question: Why did the machine prompt you to program in your weight? If you answered, "To calculate how many calories I'm burning," you are right—but what you most likely failed to consider is that the main reason it needs your weight is to calculate your basal metabolic rate.

According to calculators that determine one's basal metabolic rate (such as the one at Discovery's website: (http://health.discovery.com/tools /calculators/basal/basal.html), the basal metabolic rate of a thirty-five-year old male who stands 5′10″ and weighs 185 pounds would be 1,866.6 calories per day. The basal metabolic rate of a twenty-five-year-old woman who stands 5′4″ and weighs 120 pounds would be 1,352.7. These two individuals, then, would burn 77.775 and 56.3625 calories per hour, respectively, just to sustain their basal metabolic processes. Thus, the 300 calories burned on the treadmill are not calories burned above your basal metabolic rate; they are calories burned including your basal metabolic rate.

So, if you're the 185-pound man who burned through 300 calories on the treadmill for his one hour of effort, you burned roughly 222.225 extra calories (not 300) above your baseline metabolic rate. If you're the twenty-five-year-old woman who burned through 300 calories on the treadmill, your one hour of effort actually burned 243.6375 calories (not 300) above your baseline metabolic rate. If on the way home from your workout, you stopped off at your local Starbucks and decided that a grande-size (not venti) ice-cold Caramel Frappuccino Blended Coffee was in order—at 380 calories—you not only would have undone all of your "fat-burning" work on the treadmill but also would have added another whack of calories to your daily intake (either 157.775 or

136.3625, respectively, for the sample man and woman) that could well end up stored on your body as fat.

Think about it: if the average human body were so metabolically ineffi- cient as to burn 300 calories at the rate displayed on the exercise equipment, the species would never have survived. The calories burned in hunting and gathering would have led to death by starvation long before people could ever have found anything to eat. At that rate of calorie burn, folks would barely have enough metabolic economy to survive a trip to the grocery store. Most people have accepted blindly the information displayed on exer- cise equipment and turned exercise into a form of guilt absolution. Have dessert (600 calories of pie) and feel guilty? Just go to the health club and work on the stepper until 600 calories tick by on the screen. Beyond the fact that this seems pathetic, it just doesn't work.

Let us assume that the hypothetical man and woman have the deter- mination and time to do such a treadmill workout seven days a week. We know that if we subtract out their basal metabolic rates from the 300 calo- ries burned, they are left with 222.225 and 243.6375 calories burned. There are 3,500 calories in a pound of fat. If their appetites are not increased by the treadmill work (contrary to the norm) and they keep a stable calorie intake, it would take 15.74 days for the man and 14.36 days for the woman to burn off a pound of fat with this type of extra activity—and this is assuming that no other variables are present. Unfortunately, there is a big- time variable for which almost no one accounts: muscle loss. To exercise long enough to reach the 300-calorie mark on a stepper or treadmill, you have to perform low-intensity, *steady-state* activity.

Steady-state activity does not place a high-intensity demand on the mus- cles, which is precisely why it can be carried out for so long. Rather than engaging in a demanding use of a large percentage of your muscle fibers, you are using a small percentage of your weakest, slow-twitch fibers over and over. When you perform this type of exercise, your body can adapt by causing you to lose muscle mass—since you use such a small percentage of your muscle mass to perform this work, additional muscle is perceived by the body as being dead weight, useless and burdensome. In fact, a person who persisted in seven days per week of steady-state training could, over the course of six months to a year, easily lose about 5 pounds of muscle tissue.

Muscle tissue is the most metabolically expensive tissue in the body. You require between 50 and 100 calories a day just to keep a pound of it alive. Let's assume for a moment that it requires the lower number of 50 calories a day: were you to lose 5 pounds of muscle over time as you perform your steady-state "calorie burning" exercise on the treadmill, that would result in a loss of 250 calories per day that would otherwise be used to keep that muscle alive.

Back to our hypothetical treadmill users: the 222.225 and 243.6375 calories they burned would probably now be more like 160 and 180 calories burned, because with practice, one's treadmill economy improves and requires less effort. (Most of the perceived conditioning in steady-state activity is actually a result of the body's finding a way to make the exercise easier through improved economy of motion, and not because of improved cardiovascular condition. This is why a runner who performs another steady-state activity such as cycling will be gasping for air. As alluded to in Chapter 2, runners who train on treadmills in the winter notice a large decrease in their perceived aerobic condition when they hit the road in the spring.) So, now if we do the math for the individuals who burned about 160 to 180 calories above their baseline per day, we must subtract out 250 calories due to the loss of muscle. For all their effort, they are now a respective 90 and 70 calories in the wrong direction.

Furthermore, the production of stress hormones resulting from such overtraining also stimulates fat storage. Anyone who has attempted such a program of weight loss can confirm that you will end up feeling washed out, moody, and—worst of all—fatter. The truth is this: you cannot use physical activity to negate excess caloric intake.

MORE MUSCLE: THE REAL KEY TO BURNING CALORIES

Remember when you were a teenager and could eat everything in sight and not get fat? Somewhere in your thirties, things changed. Now it seems as if just looking at food can make you fat. What happened?

The main difference for most people is that they have less muscle in adulthood than they had in their late teens and early twenties. With aging comes a natural tendency to lose muscle, a condition called sarcopenia, as well as to be less vigorous in physical activity, which breeds further muscle loss. This loss of muscle tissue brings a sharp drop in resting metabolic rate. If you lose 5 pounds of muscle, the amount of calories you burn in a twenty-four-hour period will decrease by roughly 250 calories. While this decrease may not sound like much, it accrues over time. If you lose muscle but continue to eat the way you did when you were younger, you will gain a pound of fat in about fourteen days. Over a twenty-week period, that will end up being 10 pounds of bodyfat.

The key to getting rid of accumulated bodyfat is to get back your youthful metabolism by regaining your lost muscle mass. You have probably heard people say, "Muscle has memory," and this is one popular saying that passes the truth test. With a proper exercise stimulus, dormant muscle tissue can be reactivated to grow back to its previous size. When you regain muscle that requires 250 calories a day to keep alive, what used to be an insidious weight-gain problem will become an unrelenting weight-loss technique. As you become stronger, you will have a natural tendency to participate in more vigorous activities, and this situation will allow you to lose weight with less attention paid to calorie counting and food selection. The more reasonable your diet is, the more prone you are to stick with it. As you ride this spiral of success, you may be able to eat more like the way you did as a teenager. Putting just 5 pounds of calorie-burning muscle on your body can really turn things around for you.

PROPER EXERCISE AND DISCRIMINANT FAT LOSS

Ken Hutchins was the first person to properly explain the idea of discriminated fat loss. According to Ken, the human body can be pictured as a corporation that is run by a board of directors. A body operating on a below maintenance level of calories can be said to be running on a calorie deficit, which is like a corporation running on a budget deficit. Each of the bodily tissues can be said to represent a different department within that corporation. He then presented two scenarios:

In the first scenario, there is a budget deficit, and no department has any unusual demands. Layoffs can occur in all departments. So, the board lays off some fat, some muscle, some bone and connective tissue, as well as some nervous tissue. The corporation becomes a smaller version of its former self.

In the second scenario, there is also a budget deficit, but a large demand has been placed on the muscle department. Therefore, no layoffs can occur in the muscle department; indeed, more muscle has to be hired on. This necessitates a large layoff in the fat department. Furthermore, no cutbacks can be made in the bone and connective tissue departments, because their support is needed for the muscle department, which is not useful unless it is attached to strong bones by strong connective tissue. The recourse is that more fat has to be cashiered. No nervous tissue can be spared either, because the new muscle is also useless unless it is innervated by new nervous tissue. This imposes even more cutbacks in the fat department. With these adjustments, the corporation takes on a noticeable shape change. Under this scenario, all of the body's weight loss has been shunted exclusively toward fat loss. You have added a modest amount of shape-improving muscle and jettisoned a large amount of shape-ruining fat.

While adding muscle will raise your metabolic rate and thereby help you to burn more calories on a daily basis, if you don't also pay attention to the nutritional aspect of fat loss, it is easy to either outeat your exercise program (and thus gain fat) or select foods that will militate against your fat-loss goals. By making it a point to consume foods in their natural state, you can bring both your appetite and your fat storage down to much more manageable levels. Once this has been done and insulin levels are brought under control, it's almost automatic that nutrient partitioning occurs in a way that produces maximum lean tissue and minimum bodyfat storage.

An evolutionary gamble

To understand how to lose fat, it helps to have an understanding of why people gain fat. As odd as this may sound, it's because people have big brains. It is by pure random accident that different evolutionary branches select different adaptations to be their main tool of survival. For humans, the main tool of survival was (and is) the mind. We are the animal species that took the evolutionary gamble on a big brain, and it was a formidable gamble. What we traded off in exchange for this big brain was a greater risk of death at childbirth, owing to the fact that we give birth to infants before they are fully developed, to be able to pass a larger cranial cavity through the birth canal.

Also part of the gamble in opting for the bigger brain was that this larger brain required a constant, uninterrupted supply of energy—in the form of either glucose or ketone bodies. When this animal with the higher caloric requirements first came on the scene, and for many millennia afterward, it existed in an environment of food scarcity. To survive, it had to devise a metabolic system that could supply energy continuously to its brain, and this meant that becoming omnivorous was to its decided advantage. Developing an ability to convert protein into glucose, and to store energy (in the form of bodyfat) that could be tapped and metabolized into ketone bodies during times of caloric scarcity, bettered its chances for survival.

People get fat in modern times because, having evolved a metabolism that allows for storage of energy during times of food scarcity, the body never developed a compensatory negative feedback loop to reduce energy storage during periods of food abundance. That's because such periods never existed—until now. So, in the current environment of food abundance—particularly refined carbohydrates, which keep glycogen stores completely full (with the result that glucose stacks up in the bloodstream, raising our insulin levels)—it's a snap to store bodyfat. In the absence of a negative feedback loop, that storage never stops. Even morbidly obese people stay ravenously hungry, and they tend to be even hungrier than lean people, because they have higher insulin levels, with minimum insulin sensitivity on their muscle cells and unaffected insulin sensitivity on their fat cells. With this setup, nutrients can be partitioned directly to fat storage during periods of food abundance.

At the dawn of humanity, part of the body's normal healthful functioning involved the anabolic/catabolic cycle delineated in earlier chapters. Periods of intermittent fasting, or even starvation or food scarcity, resulted in a turnover of body nutrients that was necessary to the process of repairing and rejuvenating body tissues. As part and parcel, intermittent periods of high-intensity muscular exertion followed by periods of rest created an anabolic/catabolic cycle that allowed the body to turn over proteins within muscle tissues. Such exertion also led to intermittently emptying the muscle tissues of glycogen, so that they could maintain their insulin sensitivity and their capability to store glycogen. This waxing and waning between breaking down and building up was integral to the evolutionary development of the species. Ultimately, a metabolism evolved to store bodyfat during times of food scarcity, but now that people's big brains have solved the bulk of those food-scarcity problems, the level of obesity in Westernized society is getting out of control.

THE THERMODYNAMICS OF FAT LOSS

Losing bodyfat efficiently requires heeding the laws of thermodynamics, which means that calories must be restricted. It has often been said that "a calorie is a calorie is a calorie, no matter what its source." Many people who have disagreed with this statement have been accused of disagreeing with the laws of thermodynamics, which isn't really true: they're not disagreeing with the laws; they're *ignoring* them.

The laws of thermodynamics apply to any closed energy system, from an automobile engine to the human body. The first and second laws of thermodynamics basically state, "Energy can neither be created nor destroyed; it can only change form" and "In any closed system, the system will always progress toward entropy."[1] Stated in simpler terms, these laws are saying that you can't get something for nothing and that you can never break even. So, to counter the development of entropy within a system, energy has to be inputted to that system, and in the process of converting energy forms in order to do work, a percentage of that energy will always be lost, due to inefficiencies (mostly as heat lost into the environment).

Not being able to break even is where food consumption comes in. If you consume 2,000 calories of refined carbohydrates, the metabolic cost of processing this intake and converting it into stored energy (bodyfat) is close to zero. If you instead consume lean meats, fruits, and vegetables, the metabolic cost of converting these foodstuffs into usable energy is high. This concept is known as the "thermic cost of digestion." Consuming a diet composed of natural and unrefined foods increases the thermic cost of digestion. In addition, stable blood glucose can be achieved through gluconeogenesis—the conversion of protein, in the form of amino acids, into glucose. This conversion is a metabolically more expensive process, consisting of twenty or more metabolic steps, compared with the deep discount of consuming carbohydrates. As a result, there is a greater caloric cost to the act of simply maintaining a stable blood glucose through gluconeogenesis—that is, a backward running of the glycolysis cycle—than there is to consuming refined sugars to accomplish this same process. Moreover, consuming natural foods as opposed to processed foods will ensure that glucose levels rise and fall within the bloodstream much more gradually and thus keep overall serum insulin levels much lower.

We like to call insulin a "trump" hormone, because it trumps several other metabolic hormones necessary for fat mobilization, including glucagon, epinephrine, norepinephrine, growth hormone, and testosterone. All of these hormones are shut down by the action of elevated levels of insulin. When someone is dieting (i.e., in a calorie deficit) but is consuming a diet that is too high in refined carbohydrates, insulin levels may get to be too high, making mobilization of bodyfat difficult. A natural diet provides a double metabolic advantage in that it promotes a higher thermic cost of digestion and keeps insulin levels lower, enabling fat loss to occur in the face of a calorie deficit.

The formula, then, for optimizing fat loss from the body would be as follows:

> Energy intake − basal metabolic rate (determined largely by the degree of muscle mass) + increase because of added muscle through proper exercise + energy cost of activity, including exercise + thermic cost of digestion + heat loss to the environment = fat loss (or fat gain, if energy intake is greater than the energy cost of the listed components).

These are all elements that can be addressed in a fat-loss program, though there's no getting around the fact that calories must be restricted. If your calories are in excess of your expenditure, it's going to be a mammoth task to lose bodyfat.

INSULIN REVISITED

A prerequisite for the trainee seeking to lose bodyfat is a full appreciation of the major role that controlling insulin levels has in this process.[2] Insulin is a hormone that is produced in the pancreas. Its overall, large-spectrum function is to drive nutrient storage; its moment-to-moment function is to maintain stable blood sugar. Insulin operates by binding the receptors on the surface of cells (especially muscle cells), which creates an active complex that moves glucose from the bloodstream into the interior of the cell, where it can be metabolized.

During the evolutionary development of our species, simple sugars, which would cause rapid rises in blood glucose, were seldom encountered. In the absence of this catalyst, our ancestors' blood glucose levels were rarely elevated, even for short periods, and the cells were rarely fully filled with stored glucose. The effect was that their insulin receptors were acutely sensitive to *any* circulating insulin, since the cells typically always had room to store more glucose. Whatever glucose was stored was almost immediately turned around and used again and thus was seldom stored long term in the form of glycogen. In this environment, the body's glucose and insulin rarely, if ever, rose to abnormally high levels.

In direct contrast to those sugar-free ancestors, people now live in an environment in which simple sugars abound and are consumed routinely. As a consequence, our glycogen stores readily become full, glucose stacks up in our blood cells, and high levels of insulin are secreted. Much more glucose gets moved into the cells than can be used immediately, and the excess is packaged into long chains of glucose molecules in the form of glycogen. Once the cells become completely full of glycogen, no more glucose can be moved in. At this point, the body employs its old evolutionary trick of energy storage for use during future food shortages.

When glycogen stores are not full, glucose is moved into the cell for the process of glycolysis to take place. This twenty-step series of chemical reactions gradually converts glucose into pyruvate and then moves the pyruvate into the mitochondria. There it undergoes aerobic metabolism, which produces high levels of ATP, the basic fuel of the body. However, if the body's glycogen stores are already full when additional glucose attempts to get into the cell, this twenty-step process gets shut down three steps into the gylcolytic pathway. The enzyme at that third step then becomes allosterically inhibitive—changing shape in the presence of high levels of glucose. The process of glycolysis cannot proceed under these circumstances and instead begins to reverse into a process of glycogen synthesis. However, as the glycogen stores are completely full, the glycogen synthesis process arrests, and the glucose is instead moved toward production of a chemical called NADH, which fuels triacylglycerol (or fat) synthesis. The moral of this tale is that insulin levels have to be controlled to create a permissive environment for fat mobilization.

THE ROLE OF OMEGA-3 FATTY ACIDS

Omega-3 fatty acids, which are chains of carbon atoms linked to hydrogen, are also essential to the fat-loss process, because of their effect on hormone sensitivity. Carbon atoms can be saturated or unsaturated. A carbon atom can bind four molecules; if it binds two other carbons and two hydrogens, it's said to be fully *saturated*. A carbon atom can also develop a double bond with another carbon, so that only one hydrogen is bound to it, and that's called *unsaturated*. The position on the carbon chain where that double bond occurs gives the particular fatty acid its name. An omega-3 fatty acid has its double bond three carbon atoms back from the end of the chain, while an omega-6 fatty acid or an omega-9 fatty acid has its double bond farther back on the chain. This detail is important because the position of the double bond determines both the shape and the flexibility of the fatty acid. Omega-3 fatty acids have the double bond in a location that makes them elongated and fairly flexible, whereas an omega-6 or an omega-9, as well as a polyunsaturated fatty acid, is more tightly coiled and less flexible.

Every cell wall in the body is made up of fatty acids, the molecules of which have a carboxyl end and a hydroxyl end. One end of the fatty acid molecule attracts water and is called the "head," while the other end repels water and is called the "tail." If you drop fish oil or olive oil into water, it will form a little globule on the surface. The reason is that all the water-loving "heads" of the fatty acid will face outward toward the water environment, and all the water-avoiding tails will point toward the center, away from the water.

Recalling Figure 6.1 and the accompanying discussion, exterior to the cell wall there is water contained in the extracellular space. Interior to the cell wall there is also water in the form of cytoplasm. Every cell wall in the body is made up of a fatty acid bilayer—two fatty acids lined up tail to tail, with their water-loving heads facing out and their water-repelling tails facing in. In addition, all of the receptors necessary to maintain an appropriate hormonal balance and an appropriate hormonal response for weight loss are located on the cell membrane.

Getting the Ratios Right

If your diet is made up of natural foodstuffs that resemble a hunter-gatherer diet, you're going to be ingesting omega-3 fatty acids and omega-6 fatty acids at a ratio of roughly one to one. With this healthful ratio, a large component of your cell walls will be made up of omega-3 fatty acids and because these fatty acids are elongated and flexible, the cell walls will be fully expanded, placing all of the hormonal receptors on the exterior of the cell facing outward toward the environment, where they can appropriately interact with circulating hormones.

Straying from this hunter-gatherer ideal, if the ratio of omega-6 to omega-3 fatty acids gets to four to one, a breakdown in hormonal function begins, which can impair fat loss. Straying a whole lot further, the typical Western diet has a relationship of omega-6 to omega-3 of twenty to one. With this deranged ratio, the majority of the cell wall is going to be made up of fatty acids that are short, brittle, and less flexible. So, the cell wall will be thinner and, thus, somewhat involuted. Therefore, a multitude of the hormonal receptors necessary for fat mobilization are likewise going to be involuted—facing inward on the cell wall, where they cannot interact with their environment.

If you're attempting to lose bodyfat, all indicators point to the consumption of the appropriate amount of omega-3 fatty acids through a sensible diet. Hold up your end of the bargain by adopting this type of diet, and the hormones necessary to create the fat-mobilization process will be able to connect optimally with their receptors on the surface of the cells, allowing them to do their jobs without hindrance.

Sources of Omega-3 Fatty Acids

Omega-3 fatty acids are contained in aquatic blue-green algae and in green leafy plants and grasses, as well as in the meat of the animals that eat this vegetation. The best way to obtain an adequate supply of omega-3 fatty acids in your diet is to eat plenty of green leafy vegetables and fish. Omega-6 and other "bad" fatty acids are found mainly in grain-based agricultural products—anything derived from the seed head of a plant, as opposed to its leaves—and in the animals that eat them.

People who are attempting to lose bodyfat and are eating beef need to be aware that most of the beef supply in Western society is grain fed. For this reason, we recommend that if you are going to eat red meat, which is healthy, it should be from a grass-fed source. Humans can digest leafy green plants but are unable to digest the seed head of plants. The seed heads contain proteins that are not digestible by animals and will make them sick. This is why if you're going to eat something that's derived from the seed head of a plant, it first has to be ground into flour (or something like flour) to make it digestible. Still, these inflammatory mediators remain.

Omega-3 fatty acid sources, by contrast, are the backbone and precursors to the series 3 prostaglandins, which have a far-reaching anti-inflammatory effect. The omega-6 fatty acid sources, meanwhile, are the precursors to the series 6 prostaglandins, which are markedly inflammatory. Not only is the cell wall negatively impacted by overconsumption of omega-6 fatty acids, but also the body's inflammatory state is disrupted. It's common for people with this kind of imbalance to develop irritable bowl syndrome or gluten sensitivity. Even cattle that consume grain-based diets typically develop gastrointestinal-based disturbances; there are many more problems with E. coli contamination in grain-fed beef as opposed to grass-fed beef. Omega-3 fatty acids reign supreme in maintaining an appropriate cell wall that keeps all of the body's hormonal receptors in a position where they can best interact with their environment.

HYDRATION IS ESSENTIAL

Just as adequate hydration plays a central role in enhancing the body's response to the exercise stimulus, it also has much to do with the fat-loss process. At this point, it is useful to nail down precisely what a calorie is: a calorie is a unit of heat measurement that represents the amount of heat required to raise one liter of water one degree centigrade. So, if you were to drink three liters of ice-cold water a day, the amount of heat required to raise that quantity of water to 37 degrees centigrade (roughly body temperature) would have a thermic cost of 37 calories per liter $\times$ 3, or 111 extra calories burned per day. Such a thermic cost requires the body to burn more calories on a daily basis, and that number can grow significantly with each passing week, month, and year. Consuming cold water also lowers one's core body temperature, which again requires calories to heat the body back up to a normal temperature. The calories burned as a result of these two interrelated processes can really add up. Some researchers have suggested that drinking even two liters of ice water a day may burn as many as 123 calories.[3]

A further benefit of adequate hydration is an expansion of circulating blood volume. When you create an internal environment in which hormones are brought into play that promote fat loss, these hormones interact with the various tissues of the body, including fat cells, by being circulated. Dehydration compromises circulating blood volume and therefore severely compromises this process. When you maintain a fully expanded blood volume and adequate circulation, it is far easier to circulate all of the hormones and processed energy (in the form of ketone bodies or fatty acids, and glucose cleaved from glycogen) that aid the fat loss process.

Adequate hydration also unburdens the liver. A lot of the metabolites that accrue from fat mobilization have to be eliminated from the body. If you're adequately hydrated, these metabolites will preferentially be eliminated through the kidneys, whereas if you're in a dehydrated state, the liver is going to be charged with moving a lot of those metabolites into the bile and therefore into the stool. When you lose bodyfat, the liver is the main site where the mobilized fat is processed. If the liver is overly burdened with routine metabolic detoxification, it has less reserve for processing bodyfat. Staying well hydrated frees the liver to process mobilized bodyfat so that it can be burned as fuel.

Yet another benefit that derives from adequate hydration is improved hormonal efficiency, as proper hydration ensures that the interior of the cell (cytosol) is going to be as full as possible, stretching out so that all of its hormonal receptors are exposed to their environment, where they can interact optimally. If you're dehydrated, your hormones don't circulate as easily, and their receptors are not as well exposed.

A final benefit of adequate hydration is what we like to call *biologic reassurance*. If you spend any time watching Animal Planet or the National Geographic Channel, you will see stories about the dry season on the African plains. If you pay attention, you will come to understand this key biologic fact: drought always precedes famine. Maintaining full hydration sends a biologic message to the body that there is no threat of famine. This relationship takes on added importance when you start to restrict your calorie intake. If the body is enduring a significant calorie deficit coupled with dehydration, it perceives an urgent biologic message that there has been drought that has produced famine. This bulletin will incite the body to slow its metabolism.

Now consider what happens if there is a calorie deficit but the body is well hydrated. The state of hydration will blunt that message and minimize the risk that metabolism will slow the mobilization of bodyfat. Our evolutionary past has programmed these responses into our physiology. If people became dehydrated, their bodies reflexively slowed their metabolism and drove them to eat ravenously (if food was available) out of a fear that famine was soon to follow. Staying well hydrated tells the physiology that all is well and that there is no need to slow metabolism or raise appetite.

THE ROLE OF HIGH-INTENSITY EXERCISE

The type of training that we advocate is a dominant factor in the reduction of bodyfat.[4] We've already pointed out that steady-state exercise doesn't burn as many calories as most people believe. More important, high-intensity exercise is invaluable in the fat-loss process by helping to control insulin levels in the body. High-intensity exercise activates adrenaline to initiate a process of glycogen cleavage out of muscle cells, which is achieved via the amplification cascade that we discussed in Chapter 2. (One molecule of epinephrine will cleave tens of thousands of molecules of glucose off glycogen.) Not only is a huge amount of glucose moved out of muscle, but also the insulin receptors in muscle become more sensitive, allowing glucose to enter, and insulin levels over time will drop—a process that streamlines fat loss.

In addition, high-intensity exercise burns a respectable amount of calories during a workout and continues to burn calories, at an elevated rate, for hours afterward. Of even more value, the body's response to high-intensity exercise is to synthesize muscle, which is metabolically active tissue. A bigger muscle produces more space for glucose to enter and therefore increases insulin sensitivity. All of these goings-on are synergistic toward the process of fat loss. This series of events also explains why most men are able to lose bodyfat much more easily than most women. Men typically have more muscle mass, which means more opportunity to store more glucose in the form of glycogen, and they tend to lose their insulin sensitivity later in the process of deconditioning than do females. So, by adding muscle—whether you're male or female—you're good to go for losing fat.

Again, high-intensity exercise produces an amplification cascade for the mobilization of fatty acids out of fat cells through its action on hormone-sensitive lipase. It triggers a release of hormones, such as adrenaline, epinephrine, and norepinephrine, that act on hormone-sensitive lipase to mobilize large amounts of fatty acid out of the fat cells that otherwise would not be liberated.

A Consuming Fat-Loss Study

We conducted a fat-loss study at Nautilus North in which we put thirty-six people through a ten-week program combining diet and high-intensity training. The program required that they reduce their calorie intake by 100 calories every two weeks, starting at a below-maintenance level. Our subjects were clients aged twenty to sixty-five who had been training with us for more than a year. We tested their body composition every two weeks in a Bod Pod machine. The subjects started off with a six-set workout and trained only once a week. After two weeks, we cut their exercises back from six to four and tested them to see how they progressed.

For the first four weeks of the study, both times when we put them in the Bod Pod, we found that they lost fat—but they also lost muscle. So, we cut the subjects back to three exercises, and we noted that they didn't lose any more muscle, but they did lose fat. To test a hypothesis during weeks eight through ten, we cut the group in half, with eighteen remaining on the Big-Three workout once a week and the other eighteen performing only two exercises once a week. When we reviewed the data at the end of the study, we were surprised to see that the group that reduced the volume of their workouts to two sets once a week gained twice the muscle and lost twice the fat, on average, compared with the group that trained with three sets once a week. A workout consisting of two sets once a week outperformed a three-set workout, a four-set workout, and a six-set workout—despite the subjects' being at their lowest calorie intake during the entire program.

What we learned from this experience is that the body is adapting to everything that's going on in the person's life. People have a certain amount of adaptive energy per unit of time, and some of that adaptive energy is used in fat loss. There's a significant metabolic cost to tapping stored bodyfat, metabolizing it, and doing the necessary nutrient partitioning to make an adaptation for what is perceived as a potential starvation environment. So, this obviously consumed some of the subjects' adaptive energy, which had to be accounted for in terms of strength training and muscle gain, which was probably ratcheted down accordingly.

That's where a lot of people get into trouble. They think of exercise as something that is burning calories and fat, so when they're trying to lose weight, they ratchet up their activity levels at the same time that they're dieting. They produce too many stressors for the adaptive capabilities available and become overstressed. As a consequence, their metabolism slows, and cortisol levels spike, ultimately creating a condition in which the body becomes reluctant to let go of stored bodyfat.

—John Little

Epigenetics and the Importance of Consistency

It has long been held that genetics dictate a person's "set point" for bodyfat. According to this precept, some individuals evolved to store bodyfat more easily than others. This belief was coined the "thrifty gene hypothesis." The genotype (the exact arrangement of DNA base pairs) was thought to determine essentially everything about a person, from body shape to the way the person thinks. Now the field of epigenetics has shown that environment (especially diet) determines how the genotype will be expressed. Factors that are within a person's direct control, such as environment and diet, have been shown to have the power to alter the DNA without actually changing the genotype.[5] A person's genotype is akin to a train yard, with specific behaviors serving to flip various track switches to produce different outcomes. A person will always have the same complement of genes, but a given behavior can turn on or turn off various genes.

It also used to be thought that all of the tissues of the body cooperated for the benefit of the whole organism. Once again, epigenetics says it's not so and that different body tissues compete for resources to produce more of their particular tissue type relative to others. Accordingly, if you eat a poor diet that results in the accumulation of bodyfat, you will turn on genetic switches that propagate this process so that your fat cells can compete even more efficiently for the body's resources. These genetic switches will even alter behavior to help ensure this competitive advantage, which is one reason that it is so hard for many obese people to change to a type of behavior that sheds bodyfat.

The negative implications notwithstanding, you should be encouraged by the knowledge that you are not a slave to your genotype. Through the consistent application of sound dietary and exercise habits, you can favorably change how your genotype is expressed. Once you establish behaviors that favor lean tissue over fat tissue, you will change the competitive landscape so that being lean becomes *natural* for you. What's most amazing is that these epigenetic changes can be passed on to your offspring as if they were actual changes in your genotype. So if you become lean and strong, you increase the likelihood that your offspring will have a tendency to be lean and strong as well. Unfortunately, the opposite is also true. Another old saying is hereby born out: "Genes are the gun, but environment pulls the trigger."

A Slice of Life

I f you undertake the type of behavior that results in a hormonal balance that points to leanness, you will create a nutrient partitioning that favors lean body tissue over fatty tissue. The converse of that is also true: if you eat a lot of refined foods that are easily digestible and produce elevated insulin levels and excess storage of glycogen and bodyfat, you will lose your insulin sensitivity on your muscle cells. At the same time, insulin sensitivity on the fat cells is preserved, and you end up having nutrient partitioning that results directly in bodyfat storage. This leads to a condition known as "internal starvation." Among morbidly obese people, their entire calorie intake is shunted toward bodyfat storage.

I see this typically in my work as a physician. If I do a comprehensive metabolic panel (a panel of blood work) on these patients, I find elevated blood glucose levels, but total protein and albumin are low. (Albumin, which is a protein produced in the liver, is a marker for lean body tissue and general metabolic health.) These people are literally "starving to death" in the face of morbid obesity, because they are getting little to no value from the nutrients they are consuming. The other way I see this phenomenon in these patients is when I do CT scans, in which the images are cut in cross sections (sort of like slices of honey-baked ham). What I see are huge masses of bodyfat but also muscle tissue that is extraordinarily atrophied; I see external oblique muscles that are as thin as a sheet of paper and rectus abdominus muscles that are millimeters thin. These people are eating thousands of calories a day and are morbidly obese, but none of the lean tissue is getting fed by that intake and as a result is becoming deconditioned.

Take a tip from these patient profiles. The epigenetics of shifting your eating behavior in a positive direction will have long-term effects, beating down a new metabolic footprint for your body that is going to favor lean tissue over bodyfat.

—Doug McGuff, M.D.

SYNERGIZE

In conclusion, a trainee can do several things that, when combined, will allow for a rapidly accelerated fat-loss process.

First, eat natural, unprocessed foods. These foods typically have a lower calorie density per unit of weight. Research has shown that humans gravitate toward eating a specific weight-based quantity of food each day. In one such study, subjects were allowed to feed freely on vegetable-and-pasta salad. On one occasion, the salad was 80 percent pasta and 20 percent vegetables; on another occasion, it was the reverse: 80 percent vegetables and 20 percent pasta. On both occasions, the subjects ate almost the exact same weight of salad even though the salad that was 80 percent pasta contained twice the amount of calories as its lower-pasta counterpart.[6] In addition, unprocessed foods have a higher "thermic cost of digestion"—they require more calories to digest than processed food. Not only will you eat fewer calories per unit weight with unprocessed foods versus processed foods, but also you will burn more calories in digesting them.

Second, stay cool. Keep your thermostat down, and wear cooler clothes. This causes you to lose heat easily through your breath and skin. Remember that the process of warming your body requires heat, which, in turn, requires calories. The assets keep mounting, because even more calories must then be burned to maintain your body's core temperature.

Third, sleep well and sleep cool. Getting at least eight to nine hours of sleep per night tells your body that all is well. You're not inadvertently communicating the message to your body that it needs to be alert for predators or out scavenging. (Staying up late sends this message of searching—unsuccessfully—for food.) Sleep, particularly that obtained before midnight, stimulates release of growth hormone and testosterone and promotes cell repair, all of which is conducive to fat loss. Sleeping with the thermostat set at 70 degrees promotes deeper sleep and a decent rate of accelerated calorie burn.

Fourth, avoid stress as much as possible. It's helpful to learn stress-management techniques so that when stress occurs, you'll handle it well. Stress is interpreted in biologic terms; multitasking and worrying about inconsequential things produce a physiological state that is similar to the drought season on the African plains. If your body fears impending attack or starvation, its response is to slow metabolism and preserve bodyfat. This is true even if the stressor is just your worrying about getting off work in time to pick the kids up from soccer practice. Your body needs to get the message that all is well in order to give up stored fat easily. Stressing, particularly over minor stuff, sends the opposite message and stimulates the body to store more fat.

Fifth, employ high-intensity exercise. High-intensity training will stimulate your body to build muscle—even in the face of a calorie-reduced diet.[7] You may find that reducing the volume of your workouts during periods of reduced calorie intake will result in better progress. A Big-Three workout consisting of a leg press, seated row, and chest press, or even a Big-Two workout in which a leg press is performed along with an upper-body movement that is alternated from workout to workout (such as leg press and chest press in one workout and leg press and seated row the next), will work well. The more muscle you can build (or maintain during a calorie-reduced diet), the higher your metabolic rate will be, and the better the chances will be that all weight loss will be shunted exclusively to fat loss (rather than a combination of fat loss and muscle loss).

In the end, people will have to rely on their big brains to solve the problem of modern obesity, just as those brains once helped in addressing starvation. This does not mean that some smart scientist will come up with a solution for the masses. It means that each individual will have to understand the problem and have the discipline to apply the solution. In a world of never-ending food abundance and creature comforts, the individual must be continuously vigilant about the amount and types of food consumed and the quality of physical activity performed.

It should now be evident that the easiest way to create the calorie deficit you need for losing bodyfat is to avoid putting the extra calories in your mouth in the first place. Even a modest reduction of 150 calories per day will accrue to meaningful fat loss over time. In practical terms, the self-discipline required is much easier to summon than the effort of running on a treadmill for an hour every day (which is a losing proposition anyway). A more ambitious calorie deficit of 500 calories a day is still fairly easy to achieve. Initially, you may have to develop an awareness of counting calories, but within a few weeks, you will probably learn to manage simply by controlling the portion size of the foods you eat—and if you have added some muscle to your body, the shape change you can produce in six to twelve weeks can be amazing.

10

The Ideal Training Programs for Athletes

I f you participate in athletics, becoming appropriately physically conditioned is even more important for you than it is for your less athletic peers, because the muscle you build is going to be your major "shock absorber" and protection from injury. Part of the reason for the high volume of injuries in sports is impact trauma. It's been estimated that even jumping from a height of 2¾ feet will impart a force on the ankles of up to twenty times that of the person's body weight.[1] It doesn't take a statistician to figure out that doing this on a frequent basis is probably going to lead to something bad eventually.

PHYSICAL CONDITIONING VERSUS SKILL CONDITIONING

One of the first factors to be considered in performing any sport is the wide gulf between skill conditioning and physical conditioning. Different sports involve differing levels of complexity of skill, but all of the skills are relatively complex or else the activity wouldn't be classified as "sport" in the first place.

An article that appeared in the October 2006 issue of *Fortune* magazine titled "Secrets of Greatness" focused on how the greatest people in every field became that way. According to the article:

> . . . greatness isn't handed to anyone; it requires a lot of hard work. Yet that isn't enough, since many people work hard for many decades without approaching greatness or even getting significantly better. What's missing? The best people in any field are those who devote the most hours to what researchers call "deliberate practice." It's activity that is explicitly intended to improve performance, that reaches for objectives just beyond one's level of competence, provides feedback on results and involves high levels of repetition. For example, simply hitting a bucket of balls is not deliberate practice, which is why most golfers don't get better. Hitting an 8-iron 300 times with the goal of leaving the ball within 20 feet of the pin 80 percent of the time, continually observing the results and making appropriate adjustments, and doing that for hours every day—that's deliberate practice. Consistency is crucial. As Ericsson, a professor at Florida State University, notes, "Elite performers in many diverse domains have been found to practice on the average roughly the same amount every day, including weekends." Evidence crosses a remarkable range of fields. In a study of 20-year-old violinists by Ericsson and colleagues, the best group averaged 10,000 hours of deliberate practice over their lives; the next best averaged 7,500 hours, the next best 5,000.[2] It's the same story in surgery, insurance sales and virtually every sport—more deliberate practice equals better performance; tons of it equals great performance.

The issue included profiles of exceptional individuals in various walks of life—athletes as well as businesspeople—and they all echoed the same refrain of specific performance. An instructive example is the following excerpt on Adam Vinatieri, a placekicker for the

Indianapolis Colts and clutch postseason performer for multiple championship teams:

> [Vinatieri's] grace under pressure has earned him the nickname "Iceman." Here are his tips for staying focused while, say, 75,000 enemy fans are wishing you bodily harm, not to mention your coaches if you miss.
>
> "Stress Yourself Out." You can't expect to go out and do well when the pressure is on when you don't put the pressure on yourself. That means in practice, in the off-season, or when nobody else is there. Doesn't matter when it is; when I'm kicking I don't like to have a less than perfect day. In training, I always kick with my helmet on and buckled [team officials even pipe in crowd noise during practice]. Not everyone [works like this] but that's my signal that I'm at work and this is business. And every training kick matters just like it's a game. There should be no difference in intensity.

Vinatieri definitely knows how to perform skill conditioning. He doesn't just go out in shorts and a T-shirt and kick field goals; he tries to duplicate the conditions of a game *exactly* as they occur in competition.

Specific Practice Makes Perfect

The adage that "practice makes perfect" has merit, but it should be amended to include "only when perfectly practiced." Apart from favorable genetics, what it takes for an athlete to excel is a willingness to devote thousands of hours to the practice of a particular skill. Authorities in the field of motor learning contend that roughly ten thousand hours of practice of a particular skill is required before someone can manage to become "great" at it.[3] Moreover, the way the skill must be practiced is not merely *similar* to the way you would perform it in competition, but *exactly* as you would perform it in competition. The neural training that results in superior skill development is highly *specific*, and only by practicing perfectly will you become perfect at that skill. If you practice the skill in a way that differs significantly from the way it is performed in competition, you will not perfect that skill; you will befuddle it.

Acollegiate soccer coach in South Carolina used to come to my facility, until we had an argument over soccer balls. He believed that during soccer practice, it was a great idea to deflate the soccer balls by several pounds per inch to make them soggy. His theory was that if the players practiced with a soggy ball and could get to the point where they could kick it well, when they went into a game situation and played with a fully inflated ball, they would be able to kick it harder and farther and handle it better. He thought that this was a good way to make the inflated soccer ball feel more responsive to his players and that the difference would be to their advantage.

I tried to point out to him that the skill of handling a soccer ball is very specific and that soccer has standardized balls with standardized PSIs for that very reason. You have to practice your skill as close to competition conditions as possible, and the last time I checked, soccer wasn't played with deflated balls. The really great players—in any sport—devote thousands of hours to developing their skills with the actual items used in the game, not by changing the weight, shape, and feel of the items employed.

—Doug McGuff, M.D.

In most sports, practices and games are typically so physically demanding that they consume a significant amount of the athlete's recovery resources. An athlete who adds to this burden by then attempting to engage in conditioning exercise risks not only delaying recovery but also growing progressively weaker.

Physical conditioning

Physical conditioning is a type of training performed with the goal of improving overall physical strength and metabolic condition. It is designed to have a generalized applicability, with improvements in physical conditioning benefiting an athlete's performance in any chosen sport.

Improved physical conditioning is brought about by applying a *stressor* to the body, which it perceives as a negative *stimulus*. Acting as a biological *organism*, the body makes an adaptive *response* to that stimulus—in the form of some desired physical improvement. When performed properly, physical conditioning should not consume much time. This is because, to be productive, a stimulus must be of high intensity, and when a workout is performed at a high level of intensity, the body cannot sustain it for a long period. The goal is to incorporate the precise amount of stress that will trigger a positive adaptive response, but no more. Too much training will produce an amount of stress that exceeds the body's recovery and adaptation capacity. This *overtraining* results in weakening.

In accordance with these principles, the programs outlined in this chapter and throughout the book are of high intensity but require little time. The body is allowed to recover and become stronger, while more time is available for the other equally important part of the athlete's training program: skill conditioning.

SKILL CONDITIONING

Skill conditioning consists of the neuromuscular coordination necessary to perform certain complex motor tasks associated with a given sport—dribbling a basketball and coordinating a dunk, stickhandling and shooting, running, skating, throwing a football or a baseball, taking and receiving passes, hitting, and so on. Skill conditioning differs from physical conditioning in many ways, but the biggest way is that whereas physical conditioning has a general application to the athlete, skill conditioning has a specific application to the performance of a certain aspect of a particular sport. Soccer skill conditioning, for instance, will only improve your skills in soccer. Practicing skills outside of soccer will not help, and will likely hurt, your soccer skills.

Skills are absolutely specific. You should practice skills *exactly* as you would be required to perform them in competition. You should *not* attempt to combine (as many coaches do) your skill practice with your physical conditioning practice. For example, you should not practice with a heavier hockey puck than the one with which you play in competition. Even though the shots *feel* easier to execute when you go back to the lighter puck, you will damage your specific skills. The leverage point for maximum lift of the puck changes, and the number of motor units employed to shoot a heavier puck is different from the number required to shoot a lighter puck, so the mechanics of your shot will change. Likewise, you should not skate or run with ankle weights. The added weight will change the specific neurological pathways involved in running and skating and will confuse your nervous system.

Don't lay down neuromuscular connections that serve no purpose for the sport you are playing. No hockey federation uses a two-pound puck in its league games, no baseball league employs weighted bats, and no sport requires its athletes to play while wearing ankle or wrist weights. Get your physical conditioning in the gym using exercises that target muscle groups specifically. Get your skill conditioning by practicing exactly as you compete. Again, practice makes perfect only when perfectly practiced.

Trying to combine physical conditioning and skill conditioning is also problematic in that if you practice a skill after you have expended a high level of physical and metabolic effort to the point of fatigue, you will end up developing two skill sets: a fresh skill set and a fatigued skill set. This duality will cause neural confusion and make your performance of the skill somewhat erratic. While skill training can afford some physical conditioning benefit, that benefit is of a low order in comparison with the benefits of proper conditioning training, and the fatigue inherent in combining the activities will undermine the precise performance of the skill.

Here's the situation in a nutshell: Serious athletes have to devote a lot of time to skill training, which exacts a toll on the body's recovery resources. While skill training that is performed properly (i.e., as close to a game situation as possible) will enhance the skill set, it is usually of too low an intensity to stimulate much in the way of physical conditioning. Therefore, what's needed is a separate category of athletic training, which is proper physical conditioning. Ideally, it consists of a type of exercise that is done in a way that tracks muscle and joint function, strengthens muscles to protect the athlete from injury, and produces metabolic conditioning that the athlete can then use to advantage during competition.

HIGH INTENSITY AS THE PREFERRED MODE OF PHYSICAL CONDITIONING TRAINING

To enhance physical conditioning, competitive athletes should opt for high-intensity training as their preferred modality of exercise. By and large, this is the type of exercise that most efficiently produces generalized physical-conditioning improvements that are transferable to competition. Because athletes need time to practice the skills necessary for the given sport, and because performing the skill training during or after a physically demanding practice will only compromise the learning of the skill, the ideal physical-conditioning program for athletes is one that produces a generalized physical improvement in the most efficient manner possible.

For thoroughness and safety, it must track muscle and joint function. It must thoroughly fatigue the muscle, meaning that athletes must train to a point of momentary muscular failure to ensure the recruitment and stimulation of as many muscle fibers as possible. It must be performed with minimal rest between each exercise for optimal metabolic conditioning. Finally, it must be performed briefly and infrequently, for two reasons:

1. So that the athlete can obtain the best results from it (just as any other person does)
2. So that the athlete can obtain physical conditioning in a way that is time efficient, thus allowing more time for necessary skill practice, and that conserves recovery ability as fully as possible

RECOVERY AND THE COMPETITIVE SEASON

Coaches especially need to understand the purpose of and distinction between physical conditioning training and skill training in getting their charges ready during the off-season. Then, once the season starts, they need to continue to apply that understanding throughout the competitive schedule. Many coaches will tell their players, "The season's on, so now it's time to get serious! So, on Monday, Wednesday, and Friday, I want you in that weight room to make you stronger. On Tuesday, Wednesday, and Thursday, you're going out onto the field, so that you can work on speed and agility. On Tuesdays, you'll be doing full-pad practice. And on Thursdays, you're running patterns." This is not the best way to have athletes train during the competitive season for optimal improvement of either the athlete or the team.

A proper approach to training is not set by last year's regimen, or by a former championship team's regimen, or by tradition, or by the days of the week. A coach who fully embraces the scientific method would (and it wouldn't hurt the athlete to do so as well) first take a look at the number of games to be played and the length of the competitive season. Then, depending on the sport in question, a coach should isolate the most important competitions—such as regional or national meets in track and field or play-offs in hockey, basketball, baseball, soccer, or football. Based on where those competitions fall on the calendar, the athletes' training should be back-engineered from that competitive schedule, with the goal of timing physical conditioning workouts so that when the athletes reach these important competitive events, they are fully recovered and ready to play the game of their lives.

So many times—particularly in a sport in which athletes train themselves and in certain team sports in which players constantly seek to use what little spare time they have to improve—athletes become anxious if they aren't doing "something" in between practices. The irony is that it is during periods of doing nothing, or recovering, that all "somethings" are produced from the stimulus of training. Regardless, the athletes will typically engage in some self-directed conditioning training, often with the blessing of their coaches, when they should be recovering. They rationalize this desire to do "something" with the assertion that their competitors are doing some sort of physical exercise while they're not, so they're giving up a competitive edge. We call this the "Rocky Balboa syndrome," as it seems to factor in all of the Rocky movies at some point. Rocky is worried that his opponent is somewhere training, and unless he resorts to some daily "old-school" training methods—chasing chickens, throwing logs in the snow, chopping wood, punching sides of beef—his opponent is going to get one up on him.

This is a psychological misunderstanding of the physical processes underlying how exercise and recovery actually work. The temptation to train when they should be recovering drives far too many athletes. This proclivity underscores the importance for athletes as well as coaches of understanding the stimulus-response relationship of exercise. Guided by this knowledge, they can preview the upcoming schedule, isolate out the competition days, and then institute the proper strategy, including rest, necessary to ensure that they arrive for the event fully recovered—as opposed to becoming angst-ridden and performing a workout three or four days before the event that will leave them less than fully recovered by the day of competition.

What this means is that in a competitive season, physical conditioning workouts may need to be performed very infrequently. High-intensity workouts that are performed to positive failure to stimulate a positive adaptation may have to be postponed, owing to the energy output in games and practices. Above all, athletes should do nothing to make themselves weaker or set themselves up for a career-ending injury.

An Informal Study on the Impact of Practices and Games on a Hockey Player's Body Composition

During informal studies conducted with hockey players at Nautilus North Strength & Fitness Centre, we quickly discovered through extensive body-composition testing that any supplemental physical training performed during the competitive season yielded "zero" upside to the athlete. We first became aware of this phenomenon when one of our trainers, Blair Wilson, a genetically gifted athlete, signed with a local junior hockey team. Being a trainer, he knew about the importance of recovery, intensity, and all of those variables that affect a person's response to training.

This particular summer, since he was also an accomplished water-skier, he was performing weekly in water-ski shows and competitions. With his plate that full, he trained only infrequently, working out with weights maybe three times over the course of that summer. Nonetheless, and perhaps as a result of his intense but infrequent training, when he was about to start his hockey in September, his muscle mass was notably high.

He approached me and asked, "How often can or should I train during the hockey season?" I said in all honesty, "I have no idea, because I don't know how many games you're going to be playing, nor what your coaches are going to be having you do in your practices. Are you going to be doing 'suicides'—where you skate as hard as you can from blue line to red line to blue line? Will they be working on skills such as shooting and passing? Will they try to make your practices 'conditioning' workouts unto themselves? And then you have games throughout the season that will likewise make claims on your recovery resources." Since we were both stumped, we decided that this knowledge gap represented a ready-made opportunity to accurately measure compositional changes and see what effects practice and games had on the body composition of a hockey player.

We decided that Blair should check his body composition prior to his first practice and then every day throughout the season, to see what effect the games and practices would have. We hoped we would see a window open during the season that would allow us to train him so that he could either continue to build his strength or, at the very least, *maintain* his strength and muscle mass. Blair agreed to keep a journal so that we would know what he did the night before in practice and then, through the daily compositional testing, see what effect this had on his body.

What we soon concluded was that we couldn't train him during the season at all. From when the season started in September until the middle of December, he lost more than 6 pounds of muscle tissue. His coaches had him performing two practices a week, which then were increased to three, and he was playing one to two games every weekend. So, even the idea of a maintenance workout would have represented a "piling on" in terms of his energy output and would have caused him to lose even more muscle. If the catabolic effect of working out isn't offset by an appropriate anabolic period of rest, you begin to undermine your health.

For hockey players, a reduction of muscle means a reduction in power, strength, and the ability to resist injury. If, for instance, a groin muscle that is 100 percent recovered and maximally strong would normally tear when subjected to 100 pounds of force, that means the player is safe in encountering up to 99 pounds of force. If that same groin muscle gets smaller and weaker, that number could drop down to 60—and his chances of injury have just increased by 33.3 percent. Blair and his father, David, who is also a trainer at my facility, then began composition testing on other players on the team and noted the exact same phenomenon that Blair had experienced.

Now that the weakening effects that practices and games have on the body are evident, coaches can avoid sending their weakest team out onto the ice by incorporating sufficient rest days into players' programs so that players take the ice at their absolute strongest—and safest. What most coaches do, unfortunately, is say, "You guys were lethargic and slow in the third period of your last game. You're obviously not in proper condition, so tomorrow morning, we're going to skate you into the ground!" If the team plays poorly, it seldom occurs to the coach that the players might not be recovered from the last hard game or practice. Far from it: the team is typically subjected to a physically demanding activity, such as "suicides," that take an even heavier toll on their limited recovery ability. Eventually, the players get sick or get injured as a result of being augered into the ground by their coaches.

This is what happens if they're lucky—as a sickness or minor injury imposes much-needed rest on the players. If they're unlucky, they'll suffer a career-ending injury, one that was preventable if proper respect had been given to recovery ability and the magnitude of the toll that hard physical-conditioning practices and games take on players' bodies.

—John Little

As long as coaching practices continue at the status quo, it is incumbent on athletes to train intelligently during the off-season and to get into the best "condition" possible before they go to training camp or tryouts, or before the season starts—because *they are going to lose muscle.* During the off-season, athletes should do their best to build a muscular cushion, knowing that they stand to lose a hefty part of it during the season.

A similar prescription applies in medical therapies. It would behoove a patient who is going to be treated with chemotherapy, for instance, to build as much strength and lean tissue as possible beforehand, because once the chemo kicks in, the body is going to start consuming that muscle, and it's best that it start from as high a level as feasible. This same situation is true with sports that have a dense competitive schedule.

COMPETITION *IS* TRAINING

Competition exacts a grueling toll on the body's resources, because, from the body's standpoint, *competition is training*. In that sense, the act of competition will more specifically train an athlete for his or her skill set than just about anything else—and also provide a high degree of the necessary metabolic conditioning for specific sports performance.

In training athletes for all sorts of sports, we've observed that the metabolic conditioning they achieve while performing their sports is much like skill conditioning, in that both are exactingly specific.

The Phenomenon of Specific Metabolic Adaptation

I've trained athletes to compete in BMX using the Tabata protocol. This sprinting protocol involves twenty seconds of high-intensity sprinting followed by a ten-second recovery, and then another twenty-second sprint followed by a ten-second recovery, performed for up to five to seven cycles. The goal is to really stack lactate and push the aerobic system. From this experience, I learned right off that if the riders didn't train their metabolisms in the exact same time frame in which their specific race was performed, they would fare terribly.

The typical BMX race lasts about thirty-five seconds, maybe forty seconds on a particularly long track. What I found using the Tabata protocol is that even though by any objective measure these athletes should have been well conditioned metabolically, they crapped out about two-thirds into the race. They had become *specifically* conditioned to exert maximally for twenty seconds and then rest. When I changed the sprint protocol to a forty-second sprint followed by a twenty-second recovery, everything worked perfectly. So, metabolic conditioning is much like skill conditioning: it's very *specific*.

—Doug McGuff, M.D.

   A lot of times, the metabolic conditioning required for a specific sport can best be achieved by the performance of the sport itself or by skill practice that mimics the actual competition as exactly as possible (not physical conditioning that attempts to mimic the movements of competition), and participation in the event itself is often the best way to develop such skill sets. During the competitive season, if an athlete strength-trains at all, it should be with minimal rest between exercises to optimize the metabolic component. All the same, such training—if performed primarily with an eye toward its metabolic benefit—may not be necessary, as the athlete will be getting some degree of metabolic-training effect from participating in the sport. This type of conditioning is, obviously, ideal in that it is perfectly specific to the sport, but the strength component of training, which protects the athlete from injury and builds functional strength, will still need to be performed with a physical conditioning mind-set. This requires tracking muscle and joint function, with the intent of making the athlete stronger through the performance of three to five basic movements for overall body strength.

Sports specificity

Physically engaging in the sport yields not only a good indicator of metabolic-conditioning time frames but also the best neuromuscular training. In hockey, for instance, and this applies from the Atom level up to the professional, the typical length of a shift is forty to sixty seconds. In that span, a player has to go out and play as hard as possible and then return to the bench, at which point another line of players goes out onto the ice to do the same. The players who have just finished their all-out shift have to be metabolically recovered within roughly one and a half to two minutes of bench rest, because then they're heading back onto the ice to go all-out again for another shift. They will continue to do this for three twenty-minute periods.

In training athletes to become better-conditioned hockey players, if they're doing on-ice practicing for enhanced metabolic conditioning for this particular sport, coaches should keep the athletes at short bursts of forty seconds to a minute in length. To enhance the specificity of the athletes' metabolic conditioning, coaches should observe a game with a stopwatch in hand and isolate a particular player (or players) with an eye toward recording the pattern of exertion-to-rest. This step aids in accurately determining the optimal metabolic time frame within which to train. The knowledge gained could then be employed in practices to adjust metabolic conditioning so that it exactly tracks a player's effort-to-rest ratio during the game.

Similarly, many of the drills that hockey coaches currently employ during practices involve taking an isolated skill set out of its general context and having their players work on it in isolation. Consequently, their players develop a proficiency in performing the skill set in an isolated environment but not in a game situation. When the other contextual elements of a game are reintroduced, players are often unable to perform the skill set in the manner they exhibited in the practice setting. For the most part, the player and the coaching staff are better served by scrimmaging as though it were an actual game.

For instance, the common drills in which players pass the puck in isolation can be problematic. Passing drills in which players skate up and down the length of the ice while passing the puck back and forth to a teammate comprise a completely different skill set from passing and receiving passes during a competitive game. In addition, passing the puck in isolation eliminates the gestalt of having other players on the ice and all of the other factors inherent in a dynamic game environment. Practicing in a multicontextual environment is more likely to develop an athlete's reflexes for when and how to pass. This precept applies to all sports, and particularly to all team sports, in which the ability to anticipate the actions and reactions of others can determine a player's success as a member of a team.

To obtain the best skill and metabolic conditioning possible for players, many coaches would be better off staging scrimmages rather than practices. A coach could always have the option of blowing a whistle, stopping the play, and pointing out who was out of position and how to correct any problems or errors as they arise, as well as how those gaffes might be expressed in an actual game. There you have a teaching point that would have meaning in a game-specific vein.

This aspect speaks to specificity again in that the best practice for a particular sport is the particular sport itself. The next-best practice is doing drills that focus on specific aspects of the game and allow the athlete to develop the specific coordination of the necessary muscle groups and better neuromuscular timing. While some physical conditioning occurs as a result of these drills, most improvements are due to gains in skill. Subtle advances in body position, leverage factors, economy of motion, and technique are what really improve an athlete's speed. This is why drills that involve starts, stops, pivots, and sprints are cornerstone skills.

COACHING FOLKLORE

Most injuries in organized sports (60 percent) occur during practice, and the coaches—and many of their pregame and practice rituals—are largely to blame. One long-held and highly cherished ritual that has been shown to be without physiological purpose is stretching. It is commonly assumed that athletes should stretch for two important reasons:

1. To warm up the muscles prior to participation in the sport
2. To reduce the chance of injury during competition

No one would dispute that an athlete's muscles and connective tissues should be warmed up and that viscosity should be reduced prior to engaging in an athletic contest. However, the means to this end has been usurped by an activity called stretching—an activity that does neither of these things.

Stretching

A report issued by the Centers for Disease Control and Prevention combed through the research databases for studies that compared stretching with other ways to prevent training injuries. It combined data from five studies in an effort to identify any benefits that might come to light as a pattern. The report concluded that people who stretch were no less likely to suffer injuries (such as pulled muscles) than those who don't and that stretching did nothing to prevent injuries.[4] An even more stinging indictment came from a study of Honolulu Marathon runners, which found that stretching before exercise is *more likely to cause injury* than to prevent it.[5]

Additional articles reviewing hundreds of studies on stretching came to essentially the same conclusion: stretching does not prevent injury or muscle soreness.[6] One study oversaw a huge database of 1,538 male army recruits who were randomly allocated to stretch or control groups. During the ensuing twelve weeks of training, both groups performed active warm-up exercises before physical training sessions, but in addition, the stretching group performed one twenty-second static stretch under supervision for each of six major leg-muscle groups during every warm-up. The control group did not stretch. The researchers concluded that "a typical muscle stretching protocol performed during pre-exercise as a warm-up does not produce clinically meaningful reductions in risk of exercise-related injury."[7]

Stretching a muscle doesn't make an athlete "more" flexible either. Muscles have a limited range over which they can be stretched, which is as it must be in order for the muscles and the joints they serve to be protected. You can stretch only as far as your muscles will allow you. Attempting to stretch beyond your limitations can be dangerous, as it results in weakening of the tendons and ligaments. In a study published in the *British Journal of Sports Medicine*, the researchers concluded that the "flexibility index decreased significantly after stretching training."[8]

Since stretching does not "contract" muscles, and since contraction is what draws blood into a muscle and generates metabolic activity to provide a "warm-up," there is no warming up imparted by stretching. Again, stretching before your muscles are warmed up can actually increase your chance of injury. Putting a "cold" muscle in its weakest position (fully stretched) and applying a load of sorts (either the weight of the body or, in the case of a hurdler's stretch, muscular force) is one sure way to injure it.

A study presented at the 2006 meeting of the American College of Sports Medicine looked into what effect stretching had on strength. Strength is important in that it allows athletes to perform with greater speed and power and also protects them from injury. The study featured eighteen college students who performed a one-rep-maximum test of knee flexion after doing either zero, one, two, three, four, five, or six thirty-second hamstring stretches. Just one thirty-second stretch reduced one-rep maximums by 5.4 percent. After the subjects did six thirty-second stretches, their strength *declined* by 12.4 percent.[9] So, stretching—even for as little as thirty seconds—makes you weaker, not stronger. Since an athlete wants to be stronger and less susceptible to injury, stretching is not something in which any serious athlete should engage.

In plain English, stretching produces a weaker muscle contraction and doesn't do any of the things (from warming up, to preventing injuries, to staving off soreness, to enhancing flexibility) that it is popularly assumed to do. What it does do, in effect, is make you weaker. Having athletes engage in stretching before their practices and games accomplishes the same thing that overtraining accomplishes: sending the athlete into an important competition weaker and more subject to injury, not warmed up, and not able to generate the power that might be needed to produce a sudden burst of speed to make a play, get out of harm's way, take a more powerful shot, kick a more powerful field goal, or sprint down a soccer field. Instead, the athlete will be performing on a subpar level.

In addition, what most coaches consider to be "stretching" exercises are simply movements that create either active or passive insufficiency in the muscle groups that they believe are being stretched. How such movements can do anything to enhance muscle function is hard to fathom, because the only thing they accomplish is to place a muscle in a position of such biomechanical disadvantage that it can't actively contract, which is to say that it's doing nothing.

Cross-Training

Another myth that coaches (and athletes) need to get out of their heads is the notion of *cross-training*. The idea that practicing skills that are used in one sport will somehow improve the specific skills required for another is not at all supported by science.

The term *cross-training* was originally developed by Nike as a marketing tool to promote a particular brand of athletic footwear. It arose as a result of the injuries that occurred during the running craze of the 1970s and early 1980s when steady-state athletes were overtrained but continued to jog because they had developed an obsession with this activity. They became injured in such a way that they could not continue jogging without aggravating their shin splints (or knee or hip problems). It was also during this period that aerobic dance classes and triathlons were gaining popularity.

Against this backdrop, Nike decided to make a "cross-training" line of shoes, the concept being that you could maintain your "aerobic condition" by participating in another sport and not aggravate the overuse injury you had suffered as a result of jogging. (So, while you were allowing one overuse injury to allegedly rest, you could start working on another overuse injury in a different area of your body.) The company produced a type of shoe that could be used for running, aerobic dance class, tennis, basketball, and even weight training in the gym. It was a multipurpose shoe built into this whole notion of "cross-training," which was advanced as being a form of "active rest" (which in itself is an oxymoron) for the body and that also addressed the joggers' neurosis to constantly be doing something—in spite of their bodies' trying to warn them, "You're destroying us in the process!"

Wrapped into this concept was the belief that cross-training could also work well for skill training. This became a popular notion, particularly in sports such as BMX, where it was believed that cross-training by riding in motorcycle motocross or downhill mountain biking would produce benefits. The rationale was that when you went back to the BMX track, which is mostly a flat track, you would be moving at a lower speed. It was believed that the rider's reaction time would have been improved, and everything would appear much slower, thus improving performance, because the athlete had cross-trained by performing other similar—but different—sports. Meanwhile, all of the legitimate scientific data on motor learning clearly indicated that anything an athlete did that was similar to the current sport but not identical to it would just produce a similar skill set that runs in parallel with the real skill set required and, thus, merely confuse the skill set.

There was no need to mention any of this in a shoe manufacturer's marketing campaign, though. After all, the marketers' job wasn't selling science; their job was to address and keep alive a market that was potentially going to dry up owing to the volume of injuries that jogging had produced. They didn't want everyone hanging up those high-priced running shoes. They needed some way to keep the sales going, and the solution was this whole notion of "cross-training."

In other fields, such patently false concepts don't gain any steam. You won't, for instance, see concert pianists taking typing classes in the belief that in so doing, they will become better pianists. Athletic folklore hasn't yet permeated the world of musicians. One more time: if you want to improve your skills in a specific sport, you need to practice the skills required for that sport—period.

TRAINING THE YOUNGER ATHLETE

There seems to be a large amount of confusion about training younger children and adolescents—those aged five to fifteen. Some coaches believe that because their muscles and bones aren't fully developed, they shouldn't perform any demanding muscular work. Other coaches believe the exact opposite, that because they are young and still growing, they have a surplus of energy, and so you can work them hard with no fear of overtraining. The fact is that children can definitely be overtrained. According to statistics amassed by the National Safe Kids Campaign and the American Academy of Pediatrics (AAP):

Overuse injury, which occurs over time from repeated motion, is responsible for nearly half of all sports injuries to middle- and high-school students. Immature bones, insufficient rest after an injury, and poor training or conditioning contribute to overuse injuries among children.[10]

To this end, a proper strength-training program will benefit children of any age when it's done within reason. While children don't yet possess the hormonal environment to achieve maximal results, muscle (irrespective of the hormonal environment) always responds to loading and fatiguing with some degree of strengthening. Every child is better served by being stronger rather than weaker. In training a young athlete, or even a young nonathlete, realistic expectations must be kept foremost in mind.

In terms of metabolic conditioning for a particular sport, most children can ramp up their metabolic conditioning quickly by just playing the sport. There is no need for any strict training code to be employed with children, particularly if it's implemented in a manner that is overly intense or overly regimented and could later undermine their love for sport by being too draconian. Once the season starts and the child is playing, the child's metabolic conditioning is going to improve to the point that it needs to be. There's not much value during the season in telling a twelve-year-old, "You're going into the gym once a week." However, children can benefit from working out during the off-season just to strengthen their muscles for the season coming up the next year.

Even then, strength training for children should not be conducted with the same expectations as for an older athlete, just as your expectations for children in competition and in most other things that typically require years of practice to reach excellence need to be tailored back. Much of the intensity that is brought to children's sports activities is driven by the parents, who are trying to live vicariously through them to make up for their own perceived deficiencies. Most coaches and parents need to temper their expectations for their children and let the game be just that—a *game*.

Wanting to "pack muscle" on an eight- or ten-year-old is a misguided desire as well. Strength training is good for children and will help them somewhat, but moderation must prevail because of the child's developmental limits.

STRENGTH-TRAINING PROGRAMS FOR SPECIFIC SPORTS

The Big-Five program is an ideal physical conditioning program for most athletes, as all athletes benefit from optimal metabolic conditioning and a stronger body. While all of the body's major muscle groups are stimulated by the Big-Five workout, certain sports stress ancillary muscle groups that are not specifically addressed by the Big Five and that require specific strengthening depending on how severely they are stressed during the performance of the sport. To this end, we offer the following amendments to the Big-Five workout program as befitting athletes competing in a specific sport. As you will see, there are several exercises here that were not covered in earlier chapters; these are described after the workout.

Football

To become stronger for the sport of football, we will retain four exercises from the Big-Five baseline program, but we will break these into two workouts. Workout 1 will be followed by seven days of rest and then Workout 2 will be performed. After another seven days have elapsed, the athlete will repeat the two-workout cycle by performing Workout 1 again, and so on. The athlete should take even more time off between workouts during the competitive season.

Workout 1
1. Neck flexion/extension (anterior/posterior)
2. Lateral neck flexion (left/right)
3. Leg press
4. Pulldown
5. Chest press

Workout 2
1. Calf raise
2. Dead lift
3. Overhead press
4. Wrist curl
5. Reverse wrist curl

The additional exercises for these workouts are neck flexion (anterior/posterior), lateral neck flexion (to both the right and left sides), calf raise, dead lift, wrist curl, and reverse wrist curl. (The dead lift was described under "A Free-Weight Big Five" in Chapter 4.) The direct neck and forearm work have been added to the program owing to the inherent protective nature of those musculatures. Each of these has been incorporated on an alternating basis, so that you train your neck in one workout and your forearms in the next. Do not perform more than five exercises in total during any single workout, lest you run the risk of overtraining.

As with the baseline workout, all exercises should be performed slowly and smoothly. Move the resistance as slowly as you can without letting the movement degenerate into a series of stops and starts, and continue in this fashion until no additional movement is possible. Do not rest in between movements.

- -

The Four-Way Neck Machine

We suggest starting the workouts with neck work, so that athletes can really focus on this muscle group and train it while they're fresh. Placing neck work first in the workout will also help ensure that it is dealt with seriously. The most devastating injury that can occur from football is a cervical-spine injury with paralysis, and a strong neck is excellent protection against that. We recommend that athletes looking to build neck strength employ a four-way neck machine, such as those manufactured by MedX or Nautilus. It is important to understand the muscle action and posture required during performance to optimize the training stimulus.

As an alternative, manually resisted neck extension and neck flexion can be performed by someone with expertise, but it can be hard to do in an environment where many other athletes are working out at the same time.

—John Little

Neck Flexion (Anterior)

- **Muscle action:** The muscles that flex the neck are located on the anterior aspect of the neck and run from the clavicle to the base of the skull. All of the muscles involved in neck flexion are contained within the neck, so when performing this exercise, you want to hold your torso still and rotate only your head as you flex your neck forward.

- **Performance:** Sit in the machine facing the pads so that your nose is between the two pads. Taking hold of the handles, keep your back straight and slowly bend your neck as if you were looking down at the floor. Pause briefly in the position of full contraction, and then slowly return to the starting position. Repeat this procedure until you cannot complete a full repetition.

Neck Extension (Posterior)

- **Muscle action:** While the muscles that flex the neck forward are located on the anterior aspect of the neck and contained within the neck itself, the muscles that extend the neck on the posterior aspect (such as you would experience if you looked up above your head) have their point of origin all the way down the back to the sacrum. As a result, if you're performing your neck extensions on a four-way neck machine, you should allow for lordotic (archlike) extension of the entire thoracic and lumbar spine in order to fully involve the muscles that contract when you're extending the neck.

- **Performance:** Sit in the machine in the opposite direction from how you sat to perform the anterior flexion. This time, place the back of your head on the two pads so that the middle is your point of contact. Take hold of the handles, and position yourself forward in the seat so that your legs are almost fully extended and your buttocks are at the very edge of the seat. Slowly draw your head backward so that you are pushing the occiput (base of the skull) toward the but-

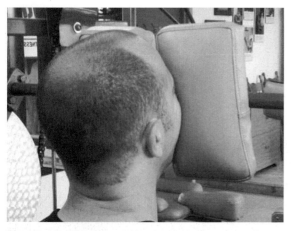

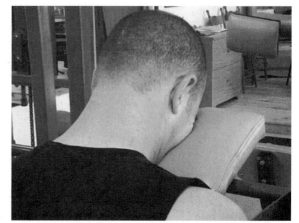

**Anterior flexion (start and
finish position)**

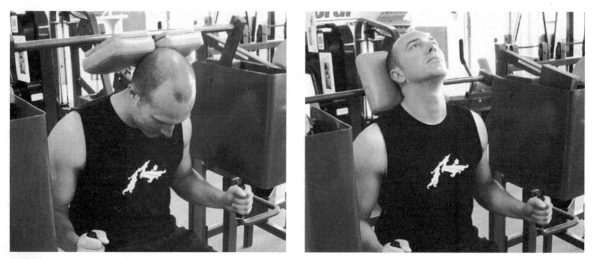

**Posterior flexion (start and
finish position)**

tocks. Also attempt to draw the buttocks toward the head by slightly arching your back as you move into a position of full contraction. Pause briefly in this position, and then slowly return to the starting position. Repeat this procedure until you cannot complete a full repetition.

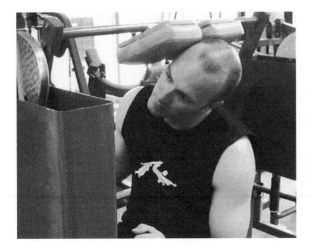

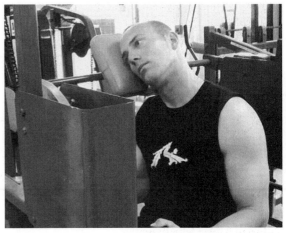

Lateral flexion, right (start and finish position)

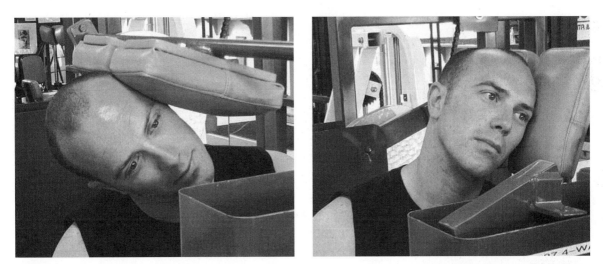

Lateral flexion, left (start and finish position)

Lateral Neck Flexion (Right and Left) The four-way neck machine allows you work the lateral aspects of the neck by simply changing your seating position. To work the right side of the neck, sit in the machine so that your right ear is aligned with the center of the two pads. Grasp the handles and, keeping your torso straight, slowly draw your head down as if you were attempting to touch your right ear to your right shoulder. Pause briefly in the position of full contraction, and then return slowly to the starting position. Repeat this procedure until you cannot complete a full repetition.

- **Muscle action:** Lateral flexion of the neck involves the anterior and posterior muscles simultaneously on either the right or left side of the neck to produce on either the right or left side of the neck to produce movement of the ear toward the shoulder.
- **Performance:** To train the left side of the neck, simply change your seat position again so that this time your left ear is aligned with the center of the two pads. Grasp the handles and, keeping your torso straight, slowly draw your head down as if you were attempting to touch your left ear to your left shoulder. Pause briefly in the position of full contraction, and then return slowly to the starting position. Repeat this procedure until you cannot complete a full repetition.

Forearm Training The following exercises train the muscles that flex and extend the wrist and contribute to a powerful grip.

Wrist Curl
- **Muscle action:** The forearm muscles that come most strongly into play when performing the wrist curs are the brachioradialis, flexor retinaculum, pronator teres, and the palmaris longus.

Wrist curl (start and finish position)

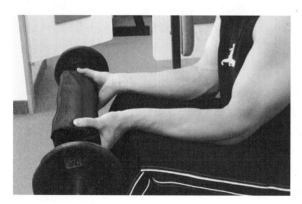
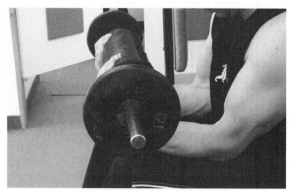

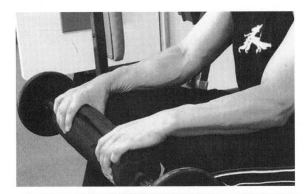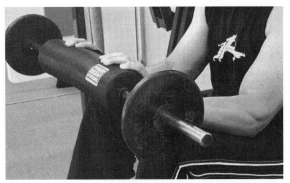

Reverse wrist curl (start and finish position)

- **Performance:** Grasp a barbell (preferably a thick bar) with a palms-up grip, and sit on a flat bench. Rest the backs of your forearms on your thighs and the backs of your hands against your knees. Lean forward slightly until the angle between your upper arms and forearms is slightly less than 90 degrees. Now slowly begin to curl your hands upward as if you wanted your palms to be facing your torso. Pause briefly in the position of full contraction, and then slowly lower your hands back to the starting position. Repeat this procedure until you cannot complete a full repetition.

Reverse Wrist Curl

- **Muscle action:** The muscles of the forearm that are most strongly involved in performing the reverse wrist curl are the brachioradialis, extensor carpi radialis brevis, extensor carpi radialis longus, extensor carpi ulnaris, extensor digiti minimi, extensor digitorum, extensor policis brevis, extensor retinaculum, abductor pollicis longus, and the anconeus (cubitalis rolani)
- **Performance:** Grasp a barbell (again, preferably a thick bar), but this time with a palms-down grip, and sit on a flat bench. Rest the bellies of your forearms on your thighs so that the front of your hands are against your knees. Lean forward slightly until the angle between your upper arms and forearms is slightly less than 90 degrees. Now slowly begin to curl the backs of your hands upward as if you wanted your knuckles to

be facing your torso. Pause briefly in the position of full contraction, and then slowly lower your hands back to the starting position. Repeat this procedure until you cannot complete a full repetition.

Hockey

The ideal workout for a hockey player would also incorporate the exercises from the Big-Five baseline program (leg press, pulldown, overhead press, seated row, and chest press) but would spread them out into different workouts with additional specific exercises for the muscles that are stressed heavily in hockey. Most hockey players will agree that the muscle groups that tend to stiffen up the most after a layoff from playing are the lower back, the adductor muscles of the inner thighs, the oblique muscles of the waist, and the buttock muscles. Because the posture for skating requires the hockey player to be bent over to some degree, there is almost a continuous isometric contraction of the lumbar muscles when you're playing hockey. These areas receive special strengthening exercises during this program, along with the adductor (or groin) muscles of the upper thighs, which are strongly involved in drawing the femur toward the midline of the body during skating; the forearms, for shooting and stickhandling; the neck, as a strong neck is protective to the player when delivering and receiving hits; and the oblique muscles, as there is a fair amount of twisting of the torso during skating, shooting, and passing. The hockey player's workout is split into four separate workouts performed on a rotating basis, with one workout performed every seven days (or even less frequently during the competitive season):

Workout 1
1. Hip and back machine
2. Seated row
3. Overhead press
4. Adduction machine
5. Rotary torso

Workout 2
1. Leg press
2. Pulldown

3. Chest press
4. Wrist curl
5. Reverse wrist curl

Workout 3

1. Lower-back machine
2. Seated row
3. Overhead press
4. Adduction machine
5. Rotary torso

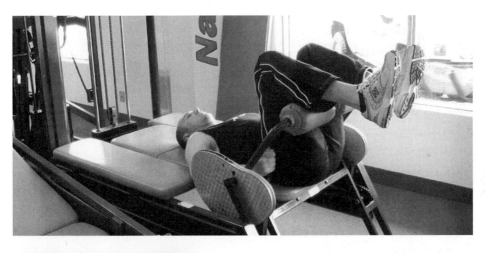
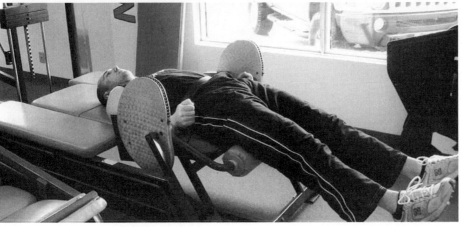

Hip and back machine (start and finish positions)

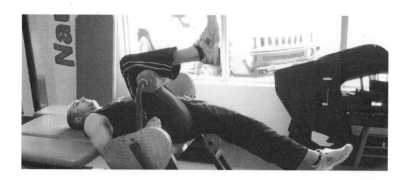

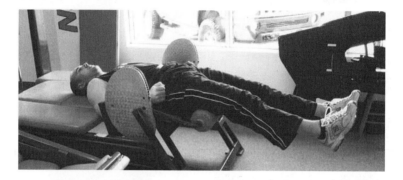

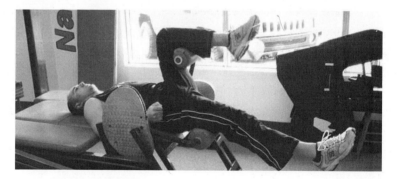

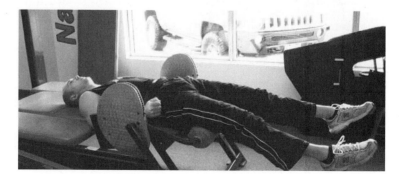

**Hip and
back machine**

Workout 4

1. Neck flexion (anterior/posterior)
2. Lateral neck flexion (left/right)
3. Leg press
4. Pulldown
5. Chest press

Perform one workout every seven days (or less frequently during the competitive season), starting with Workout 1. The next week, you would perform Workout 2; the following week, you would perform Workout 3; and after that week, you would perform Workout 4. After another seven days (or longer), you would rotate through the four-workout cycle again. The exercises not covered previously should be performed as follows:

Hip and Back Machine
- **Muscle action:** All jumping, thrusting, and skating motions (particularly when power is required) rely strongly on involvement of the gluteus maximus (buttock) muscles.
- **Performance:** Lie down on the pad on the hip and back machine and position your body so that your hips are aligned with the axis of the two cams. Extend both legs while pushing back with your arms until your legs, with the feet together, are locked at the knees and below parallel to the floor, so as to arch the back. Pause briefly in this position of full muscular contraction. Hold one leg locked at full extension, and then allow the other leg to come back as far as possible until the extended leg cannot remain still. Slowly push that leg back out until both legs are joined at extension. Arch your back and contract your buttocks. Repeat with the other leg. Continue in an alternating fashion until a full repetition cannot be completed.

Adduction Machine
- **Muscle action:** The adductor muscles of the inner thighs are involved whenever the leg is drawn toward the midline, such as during crossovers in skating.
- **Performance:** Sit in the adductor machine and place your knees and ankles on the movement arms in a spread-legged position. Your inner

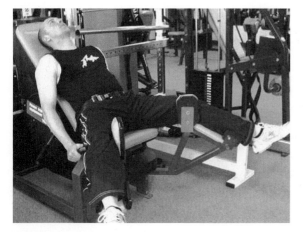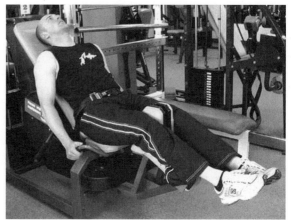

Nautilus adduction (start and finish position)

thighs and knees should be firmly against the resistance pads. Adjust the lever so that there is resistance in the position of full extension. Keeping your head and shoulders against the seat back, slowly pull your knees and thighs toward each other until they are smoothly together. Pause in the knees-together position briefly before slowly allowing your legs to return to the stretched position. Repeat the procedure until a full repetition cannot be completed.

Rotary Torso

■ **Muscle action:** This movement strongly involves the external and internal oblique musculature on either side of the waist. Their function is to bend the spine to the side and to rotate the torso, such as when an athlete takes a shot in hockey, swings a bat or throws a ball in baseball, or swings a club in golf.

■ **Performance:** Sit upright in the machine on either the right or left side. If you're starting from the right, sit in the machine with your lower legs crossed and to the right of the pad. This will secure your lower body, thus ensuring that all of the motion in the exercise will be produced by the muscles that rotate the trunk (the oblique muscles). Rest your arms on the pads and take hold (one in each hand) of the two vertical bars. You should be sitting up straight so that your nose is centered between the bars (sustain this position throughout the move-

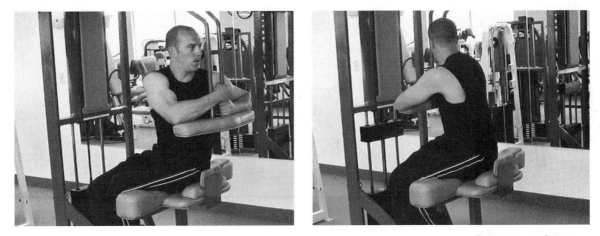

Rotary torso (start and finish position)

ment). Slowly begin to twist your torso to the right (toward the weight stack). Keep your back as straight as possible during the movement and your nose centered between the bars. When you have reached a position of full contraction, pause briefly, and then lower slowly back to the starting position, making sure not to let the weights touch the stack (which will unload the musculature) as you do so. Continue to twist to the right and return under control until you can no longer complete a full repetition. Upon completion, exit the machine and reenter it from the left side. Repeat the procedure for the muscles on the left side of your torso in the same manner that you did for your right side.

Baseball

Most of the exercises in the football-training program apply to a baseball player's strengthening program. However, given the muscular structures involved in throwing, some specific training for the musculature of the shoulders and the oblique muscles on either side of the waist is called for.

Workout 1
1. Leg press
2. Pulldown
3. Chest press

4. Lateral raise
5. Rear deltoid

Workout 2
1. Calf raise
2. Shrug
3. Rotary torso
4. Wrist curl
5. Reverse wrist curl

Baseball players should alternate between the two workouts, with seven days in between each workout.

Rear Deltoid
- **Muscle action:** The rear deltoid serves to draw the arm back behind the body, such as when an athlete pulls his arm back to throw a ball.
- **Performance:** This is another exercise in which a Nautilus machine is preferred. Sit in the machine so that your back is resting on the back pad. Place your elbows on the pads in front of you so that your upper arms are at 90 degrees to your torso. Slowly begin to draw your upper arms back until they are behind your torso. Pause in the position of full contraction, and then slowly let your arms return to the stretched (or starting) position. Repeat in this fashion until you can no longer complete a full repetition.

Golf
In addition to general overall strength, a golfer should pay attention to the forearm and oblique musculatures. For this reason, we suggest performing the following two workouts on an alternating basis once every seven days:

Workout 1
1. Leg press
2. Seated row

3. Chest press
4. Wrist curl
5. Reverse wrist curl

Workout 2
1. Calf raise
2. Lower-back machine
3. Pulldown
4. Overhead press
5. Rotary torso

ENDGAME

The foregoing programs are more than sufficient to build an athlete's strength up to its maximum level. Do not add any exercises into these programs, as they should never exceed five per workout to ensure that the athlete is giving 100 percent to each exercise, each and every workout. An athlete who performs one of these workouts should be able to engage in skill training within two days. The day after the strength workout, however, would be better spent relaxing and reviewing competitive data, such as watching videos of the last game or competitive event.

One point we want to make in closing out this chapter is that both physical training and skill training are important, but from a more aerial view, the genetic factor is a major determinant of an athlete's success and dominance. You can become a good athlete through proper skill conditioning and physical conditioning, but becoming a truly great, world-class athlete _requires_ _proper_ _skill_ and _physical_ _conditioning_—and _genetics._ At the highest levels of competitive sports—collegiate football, professional football, hockey, baseball, soccer, golf, and the like—a lot of ridiculous folklore has come out of the coaching world because these coaches have been given athletes who have benefited from a vicious natural-selection process. [These genetically gifted individuals could train in almost any fashion and still show outstanding results.]

Unfortunately, most people do *not* share in these genetic gifts. As a consequence, poor training practices that are better tolerated by the genetically gifted athlete reinforce primitive, superstitious coaching folklore. A rational analysis of dynamic winning teams would tip the scales of attribution for their success in favor of their scouts—not their coaches. Talent scouting is the thing that makes an outstanding team. If you can skim the cream of the genetic crop to build your team, then the odds are that you will have a winning team. If ideal genetics is combined with an ideal, scientifically sound training program such as the ones in this chapter, athletic success is sure to follow.

The Ideal Training Program for Seniors

O n the subject of exercise requirements, senior citizens need to let go of the idea that somehow they're different from the rest of the population because of their age. Being older doesn't change much of anything on that front. All of the physiological mechanisms necessary for the human body to produce a physiological adaptation to the exercise stimulus remain intact through every stage of life. The only meaningful difference that pertains from a physiological standpoint with regard to older people versus younger people is that the older population has had more time for the deconditioning process to do its damage. They have dug a deeper decompensatory hole, metabolically speaking, than the average younger person who is embarking on a resistance-training program.

Consider the physiological constitution of the average thirty-five-year-old man who has never trained with weights. He is right at the threshold where he will spontaneously start to lose a significant amount of lean mass unless an appropriate muscle-strengthening stimulus intervenes. A similar situation occurred with the average seventy-year-old man when he was thirty-five—but has continued unchecked for the ensuing thirty-five years. The senior citizen is starting from a point of worsened muscular condition because he has allowed the process of degradation (or atrophy) of his muscular system to take place without remedy for a much longer time.

Nevertheless, for both individuals, the remedy and the physiological mechanism that needs to be engaged to reverse the process of atrophy are the same. The precautions that need to be taken in training are also the same for any member of the population—though with seniors, strict adherence is essential. This mandates that seniors perform biomechanically correct exercise through a full range of motion that is tolerated by the body. Also, the exercise must be done in a way that properly tracks muscle and joint function. Most important, any exercise must be performed in a manner that properly controls the forces brought to bear on muscles, joints, and connective tissues so that the chances of injury are obviated as fully as possible. Again, all of the guidelines that apply to younger people and exercise also apply to seniors, only more so.

The senior population has the most to gain from a high-intensity strength-training program.

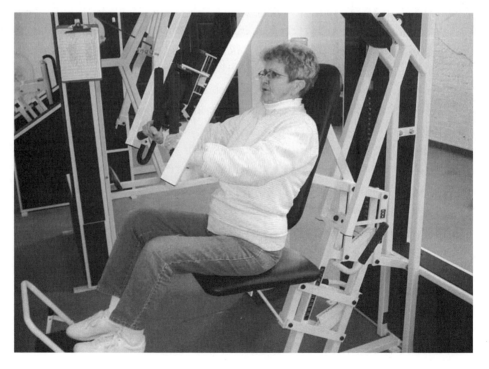

In our facilities, all of the managers and instructors on staff are careful with everyone we train, and seniors are not a de facto exception in any way. In general, the only time it's necessary to modify a given training program is when a client (and this again applies across the board) has an injury or a condition such as arthritis that might call for limiting the range of motion initially. This might mean changing the machine setup to a minor extent, but in terms of how we apply the exercise protocol, there is not (nor should there be) any difference.

THE BENEFITS OF STRENGTH FOR SENIORS

The benefits attainable from strength training are even more compelling for senior citizens than for others, just by virtue of the fact that seniors have so much more that they can gain back.[1] In case after case, when a proper training stimulus is applied to the physiology of elderly people, the rate at which they strengthen is astounding. It doesn't take a lot of stimulus for them to get back to a normal baseline, because their muscles have, in effect, been lying dormant, desperate for a stimulus to awaken and reactivate them. It is not uncommon to see a doubling of strength (yes, a 100 percent increase) in as little as six to twelve weeks. This is the metabolic equivalent of "coming back from the dead" in terms of how much a person's body—and vitality—can change.

Studies have revealed that, for seniors, a proper strength-training program can produce the following changes in the muscle and in the health benefits that attend having more muscle:

- Regained muscle strength and function[2]
- Increased muscle strength and muscle size in senior men and women, including nursing home residents[3]
- Enhanced walking endurance[4]
- Reduced bodyfat levels[5]
- Increased metabolic rate[6]
- Reduced resting blood pressure[7]
- Improved blood lipid profiles[8]
- Increased gastrointestinal transit speed[9]

- Enhanced glucose utilization[10]
- Alleviated low-back pain[11]
- Increased bone mineral density[12]
- Eased arthritic discomfort[13]
- Relieved depression[14]
- Improved postcoronary performance[15]

It's also noteworthy that not one of these studies reported any training-related injuries.

The exothermic benefit of muscle

Another important consideration for seniors is that muscle regulates body temperature. The body is supposed to maintain an internal temperature of 98.6 degrees, but as people lose muscle over the years, they also lose the heat that muscle provides. As a result, they tend to become more vulnerable to both hot and cold, which causes unhealthful fluctuations in body temperature. This condition can be a serious problem with elderly people, particularly if they become sick.

Doctors know that most people who get pneumonia or a urinary tract infection will develop a fever, but not elderly patients. More often than not, the elderly patient under such circumstances is hypothermic. The reason is that muscle generates considerable heat, because the metabolic activity of the body, as with all energy activity that is governed by thermodynamics, is exothermic, meaning that it produces heat. In a car, for instance, the engine produces significant amounts of heat. That's why car manufacturers install radiators. Remember the first law of thermodynamics, which says, in effect, that you can't get something for nothing. Energy always has to be inputted into the system. The second law of thermodynamics says, in effect, that you can never break even. This means that as energy is being converted, it is always wasted external to the system. This is precisely how body heat is produced; it is the product of the mechanical inefficiency of energy consumed by muscle tissue. If your body doesn't have an adequate supply of muscle tissue, you will not produce enough heat so that the excess can be used to maintain your body's temperature.

Most people don't realize how vulnerable elderly people are to hypothermia. An elderly person who happens to slip and fall in the shower and is not discovered for several hours is as likely to die from hypothermia as from any other consequence of the fall. Muscle, we repeat, is a vital protective tissue for the elderly population. The more of it, the better.

The dozen-plus benefits listed in the preceding section are not so much direct effects of strength training as they are indirect effects that evolve as the body produces or restores more muscle. In the case of arthritis, an arthritic joint is going to move more efficiently if a strong muscle is controlling it, rather than a weak muscle. With regard to osteoporosis, studies show a benefit from strength training among seniors when the weight is significant: 75 to 80 percent of a subject's one-rep maximum. Anything less than this will probably be insufficient load to stimulate the body to make changes in bone mineral density. With senior citizens, as with everyone else, a proper strength-training program must use a meaningful load and attempts should always be made to progress that load as the trainee's strength increases over time.

This is why the approach of most fitness professionals to treat senior citizens as though they were pieces of fine porcelain is detrimental. Yes, caution must be exercised with the senior trainee. Care must be taken in the way the exercise is administered, such as in the control of movement speed and the diminishing of momentum, so that forces into joints are controlled—but this is true of all trainees. Trainees and trainers can't be namby-pamby about selecting weights or allowing for exertion of energy. If a "toned-down" approach is employed, the roster of benefits either will be diminished or will not be forthcoming at all.

MEDICINAL IMPACT

Strength training is the best preventive medicine in which a human being can engage. In many instances, senior citizens are being medicated to improve those listed biomarkers of health, never having been told that it is fully within their power to achieve these same effects through proper resistance training. Many of the metabolic benefits that increase in tandem with an increase in muscle can obviate the need for the medications that seniors commonly ingest to treat the symptoms of such complications as high (or low) blood pressure and high cholesterol levels.

Seniors (or anyone else) who engage in a proper strength-training program and who are on medication to treat the symptoms of such conditions as diabetes should be closely monitored, as their medication may well have to be reduced. Recall the amplification cascade from Chapter 2. If, for instance, a senior with non-insulin-dependent diabetes is prescribed oral hypoglycemics, when the glycogen mobilization cascade occurs during workouts, insulin sensitivity will improve significantly along with gains in strength and muscle mass. The consequence of dosing an oral hypoglycemic agent that is *just adequate* for the senior at one point is that six to twelve weeks into a strength-training program, the improvement in insulin sensitivity may cause the blood sugar to fall too low.

A similar situation exists for blood pressure medication. Strength training produces more muscle mass—and more growth of vascular tissue to support it. As a trainee generates more blood vessels to supply the newly growing muscle, the vascular bed total volume enlarges, and the peripheral vascular resistance will start to decrease. So, for trainees who take blood pressure medicine or antihypertensives, the dose that was just adequately controlling their blood pressure is now making them hypotensive and light-headed. Strength training is in itself "strong medicine" that stimulates the body to produce powerful results.

INDEPENDENCE AND LIBERTY

Above and beyond all of the previously described benefits that a proper strength-training program affords is the opportunity for senior citizens to reclaim their independence and liberty. A recent study conducted by physiologist Wayne Wescott took nonambulatory seniors from a nursing home and had them participate in a brief workout involving one set of six different exercises for a fourteen-week period. The average age of the subjects was eighty-eight and a half. At the end of the study, the seniors had averaged a four-pound gain in muscle, a three-pound loss of fat, an increase in strength of more than 80 percent in their lower-body musculature, and an increase in strength of almost 40 percent in their upper-body muscu-lature. They improved their hip and shoulder flexibility by an average of 50 percent and 10 percent, respectively. More important, at the end of the study, many of the formerly wheelchair-bound subjects were able to walk again. They were out of their wheelchairs and no longer required around-the-clock nursing.[16]

The ability to get around and do things for oneself defines independence, particularly in old age. Engaging in a brief and basic strength-training pro-gram can restore to seniors a measure of independence and dignity that they had enjoyed in earlier years but that had gradually diminished as they allowed their muscles to atrophy. It can be a brand-new lease on life.

You've probably seen the television commercials for electric wheelchairs and scooters targeted to seniors as a means of expanding their mobility. These devices are fine as far as they go, but they can never restore lost mobility. They may allow people access to more location options than they would otherwise have, but many routine activities still will require outside assistance. Having to constantly depend on the kindness of others puts people in a vulnerable position, physically as well as psychologically.

Today's elderly people in particular belong to a generation accustomed to being active. So, typically, as soon as they regain the capability to be active, they *become* active again. It is not necessary for seniors to be on a "walking program" or on a treadmill or exercise bike for them to get suffi-cient levels of activity. When senior citizens become stronger, their activity levels will rise as a matter of course. From a cosmetic perspective, every-thing improves, including their appearance, their posture, their demeanor, and their skin tone. As the senior's level of muscle mass increases, every-thing else tracks along with it.

THE SENIOR'S BIG-THREE WORKOUT

As a rule, senior citizens should perform the same baseline program as anybody else. Then again, there are bound to be exceptions. For those who find the program too taxing, we've had good results with trainees who per-form no more than three exercises in a given workout. Here's an example:

1. Seated row
2. Chest press
3. Leg press

Many of these same seniors train no more frequently than once every seven to fourteen days. Don't worry that this is "not enough." It is. If you think of an elderly person as someone trapped inside his or her body with diminished mobility, then it follows that as soon as enough strength has been produced to restore mobility, the person's activity levels are going to increase simultaneously.

In summary, we recommend the basic Big-Five routine outlined in Chapter 4 as an ideal training program for senior citizens. However, if mobility issues or other factors preclude that approach, doing a basic Big-Three routine and aggressively focusing on progression on these basic movements will get the average senior citizen a lot of bang for the metabolic buck.

A REVOLUTIONARY STUDY

In closing, we would like to share with you a study that can only be described as "revolutionary" in its impact in regard to strength training and senior citizens. As unlikely as this may sound, it revealed that strength training can actually reverse the aging process.

For the study, the results of which were was published in the online medical journal *Public Library of Science*, researchers recruited twenty-five healthy seniors (average age seventy) and an equal number of college students (average age twenty-six). All of the subjects submitted to having muscle biopsies performed, and 24,000 genes were compared for each participant. It was noted that 600 genes were markedly different between the older and younger subjects. Prior to the study, the senior and younger groups were found to have similar activity levels, though the young people, as one might expect, were considerably stronger than their older counterparts. The seniors then took part in a strength-training program for six months. Afterward, the researchers found that the seniors had gone from being 59 percent weaker than the young adults to being only 38 percent weaker. More important was the change in the seniors' genes. The gene-expression profile (or genetic fingerprint) of the seniors changed noticeably, looking a lot more like that of the younger trainees. The researchers concluded their study by stating:

> Following exercise training the transcriptional signature of aging was markedly reversed back to that of younger levels for most genes that were affected by both age and exercise. We conclude that healthy older adults show evidence of mitochondrial impairment and muscle weakness, but that this can be partially reversed at the phenotypic level, and substantially reversed at the transcriptome level, following six months of resistance exercise training.[17]

Nothing else in human history has shown a functional reversing of age in humans at a molecular level. When the drug Resveratrol was shown to produce *some* reversal of aging in mice and worms, it flew off the shelves as an age-reversal agent—without any proof that it had a similar effect in humans. Now here, after *millennia* of searching for the "fountain of youth"—anything that might extend life or objectively reverse aging in humans, going back as far as our earliest recorded literature in *The Epic of Gilgamesh*—a clinical study has essentially said, "Look, here it is—an actual functional reversal of aging at the molecular level!" It is astounding that genes that were functioning poorly at an elderly level could be returned to a normal level of functioning in elderly people.

But it's not surprising to us, nor to anyone who performs the type of training that we advocate. It's not unusual to see an elderly person start working out with minimal weights and then, in a short span of time, see the person's strength be equal to or greater than that of the average twenty-five-year-old. We have seventy-five- and eighty-year-old clients training at our facilities, and routinely when we bring in a new twenty-five-year-old client, the weights at which we start the young adult do not approach what most of our older established clients are currently using.

Having said this, the most amazing thing that happened after this study came out in 2007 was—*nothing*. That news of this magnitude should come out during our lifetimes and not be on the front page of every newspaper and on every evening news program was inexplicable to us. Perhaps it failed to garner much attention because people are more than willing to take a pill, thinking it's going to reverse their aging, and it's only the exceptional individual who would hear such news and say, "I can do something for myself, by the sweat of my own brow; by applying my own effort and my own work ethic, I can achieve this for myself!" Perhaps.

For this benefit to occur, an individual of any age must be willing to train with effort, a rare find in our society. The beautiful thing is that the ones who understand and apply this principle are the ones with whom we get to work—and the ones who are reaping all the benefits we've covered in this book.

Notes
The Scientific Literature Supporting
Body by Science

Introduction

1. U.S. Department of Commerce, Bureau of the Census, *Historical Statistics of the United States*; and Department of Health and Human Services, *National Center for Health Statistics Reports* 54, no. 19 (June 28, 2006), dhhs.gov.

2. P. S. Bridges, "Prehistoric Arthritis in the Americas," *Annual Review of Anthropology* 21 (October 1992): 67–91; A. Liverse et al., "Osteoarthritis in Siberia's Cis-Baikal: Skeletal Indicators of Hunter-Gatherer Adaptation and Cultural Change," *American Journal of Physical Anthropology* 132, no. 1 (2007): 1; P. S. Bridges, "Vertebral Arthritis and Physical Activities in the Prehistoric Southeastern United States," *American Journal of Physical Anthropology* 93, no. 1 (1994): 83; W. J. MacLennan, "History of Arthritis and Bone Rarefaction on Evidence from Paleopathology Onwards," *Scottish Medical Journal* 44, no. 1 (February 1999): 18–20; and P. S. Bridges, "Degenerative Joint Disease in Hunter-Gatherers and Agriculturists from the Southeastern United States," *American Journal of Physical Anthropology* 85, no. 4 (August 1991): 379–91.

Chapter 1

1. W. C. Byrnes, P. McCullagh, A. Dickinson, and J. Noble, "Incidence and Severity of Injury Following Aerobic Training Programs Emphasizing Running, Racewalking, or Step Aerobics," *Medicine and Science in Sports and Exercise* 25, no. 5 (1993): S81.

2. Plutarch, *Lives, vol. II, translated from the Greek, with Notes* and *A Life of Plutarch*, by Aubrey Steward and George Long (London: George Bell and Sons, 1899), 46–47.

3. Herodotus, *The History of Herodotus*, 3rd edition, translated by G. C. Macaulay (London: MacMillan and Co., Limited, 1914), 96, 105–6.

4. Lucian, "Pro Lapsu inter Salutandum," in *The Works of Lucian of Samosata (Vol. III)*, translated by H. W. Fowler and F. G. Fowler (Oxford: The Clarendon Press, 1905), 36.

5. G. Whyte, "Is Exercise-Induced Myocardial Injury Self-Abating?" *Medicine and Science in Sports and Exercise* 33, no. 5 (May 2001): 850–51, "Echocardiographic Studies report cardiac dysfunction following ultra-endurance exercise in trained individuals. Ironman and half-Ironman competition resulted in reversible abnormalities in resting left ventricular diastolic and systolic function. Results suggest that myocardial damage may be, in part, responsible for cardiac dysfunction, although the mechanisms responsible for this cardiac damage remain to be fully elucidated"; W. L. Knez et al., "Ultra-Endurance Exercise and Oxidative Damage: Implications for Cardiovascular Health," *Sports Medicine* 36, no. 5 (2006): 429–41; J. E. Sherman et al., "Endurance Exercise, Plasma Oxidation and Cardiovascular Risk," *Acta Cardiologica* 59, no. 6 (December 2004): 636–42; and R. Shern-Brewer et al., "Exercise and Cardiovascular Disease: A New Perspective," *Arteriosclerosis, Thrombosis, and Vascular Biology* 18, no. 7 (July 1998): 1181–87.

6. D. R. Swanson, "Atrial Fibrillation in Athletes: Implicit Literature-Based Connection Suggests That Overtraining and Subsequent Inflammation May Be a Contributing Mechanism." *Medical Hypotheses* 66, no. 6 (2006): 1085–92.

7. M. Deichmannet, A. Benner, N. Kuner, J. Wacker, V. Waldmann, and H. Naher, "Are Responses to Therapy of Metastasized Malignant Melanoma Reflected by Decreasing Serum Values of S100β or Melanoma Inhibitory Activity (MIA)?" *Melanoma Research* 11, no. 3 (June 2001): 291–96, "In metastatic melanoma S100β [a marker of cancer] as well as melanoma inhibitory activity (MIA) are elevated in the serum in the majority of patients. Elevation has been found to correlate with shorter survival, and changes in these parameters in the serum during therapy were recently reported to predict therapeutic outcome in advanced disease"; and R. V.

T. Santos, R. A. Bassit, E. C. Caperuto, and L. F. B. P. Costa Rosa, "The Effect of Creatine Supplementation upon Inflammatory and Muscle Soreness Markers After a 30km Race," *Life Science* 75, no. 16 (September 15, 2004): 1917–24, "After the test (a 30km run), athletes from the control group presented an increase in plasma CK (4.4-fold), LDH (43%), PGE2 6.6-fold) and TNF-alpha [another marker of cancer] (2.34-fold) concentrations, indicating a high level of cell injury and inflammation."

8. H. J. Wu, K. T. Chen, B. W. Shee, H. C. Chang, Y. J. Huang, and R. S. Yang, "Effects of 24 H Ultra-Marathon on Biochemical and Hematological Parameters," *World Journal of Gastroenterology* 10, no. 18 (September 15, 2004): 2711–14, "Results: Total bilirubin (BIL-T), direct bilirubin (BIL-D), alkaline phosphatase (ALP), aspartate aminotransferase (AST), alanine aminotransferase (ALT) and lactate dehydrogenase (LDH) increased statistically significantly ($P<0.05$) the race. Significant declines ($P<0.05$) in red blood cell (RBC), hemoglobin (Hb) and hematocrit (Hct) were detected two days and nine days after the race. 2 days after the race, total protein (TP), concentration of albumin and globulin decreased significantly. While BIL, BIL-D and ALP recovered to their original levels, high-density lipoprotein cholesterol (HDL-C) remained unchanged immediately after the race, but it was significantly decreased on the second and ninth days after the race. Conclusion: Ultra-marathon running is associated with a wide range of significant changes in hematological parameters, several of which are injury related. To provide appropriate health care and intervention, the man who receives athletes on high frequent training program high intensity training programs must monitor their liver and gallbladder function." [Note: HDL is lowered, LDL is increased, red blood cell counts and white blood cell counts fall. The liver is damaged and gall bladder function is decreased. Testosterone decreases.]

9. M. J. Warhol, A. J. Siegel, W. J. Evans, and L. M. Silverman, "Skeletal Muscle Injury and Repair in Marathon Runners After Competition," *American Journal of Pathology* 118, no. 2 (February 1985): 331–39, "Muscle from runners showed post-race ultrastructural changes of focal fiber injury and repair: intra and extracellular edema with endothelial injury; myofibrillar lysis, dilation and disruption of the T-tubule system, and focal mitochondrial degeneration without inflammatory infiltrate (1–3 days). The mitochondrial and myofibrillar damage showed progressive repair by 3–4

weeks. Late biopsies showed central nuclei and satellite cells characteristic of the regenerative response (8–12 weeks). Muscle from veteran runners showed intercellular collagen deposition suggestive of a fibrotic response to repetitive injury. Control tissue from non-runners showed none of these findings."

10. J. A. Neviackas and J. H. Bauer, "Renal Function Abnormalities Induced by Marathon Running," *Southern Medical Journal* 74, no.12 (December 1981): 1457–60, "All post race urinalyses were grossly abnormal. . . . We conclude that renal function abnormalities occur in marathon runners and that the severity of the abnormality is temperature-dependent."

11. M. K. Fagerhol, H. G. Neilsen, A. Vetlesen, K. Sandvik, and T. Lybert, "Increase in Plasma CalProtectin During Long-Distance Running," *Scandinavian Journal of Clinical and Laboratory Investigation* 65, no. 3 (2005): 211–20, "Running leads to biochemical and hematological changes consistent with an inflammatory reaction to tissue injury. . . . During the marathon, half-marathon, the 30-km run, the ranger-training course and the VO_2 max exercise, calprotectin levels increased 96.3-fold, 13.3-fold, 20.1-fold, 7.5-fold and 3.4-fold, respectively. These changes may reflect damage to the tissues or vascular endothelium, causing microthrombi with subsequent activation of neutrophils."

12. $S100\beta$ is a protein that reflects central nervous system injury. N. Marchi, P. Rasmussen, M. Kapural, V. Fazio, K. Kight, A. Kanner, B. Ayumar, B. Albensi, M. Cavaglia, and D. Janigro, "Peripheral Markers of Brain Damage and Blood-Brain Barrier Dysfunction," *Restorative Neurology and Neuroscience* 21, no. 3–4 (2003): 109–21, "$S100\beta$ in serum is an early marker of BBB openings that may precede neuronal damage and may influence therapeutic strategies. Secondary, massive elevations in $S100\beta$ are indicators of prior brain damage and bear clinical significance as predictors of poor outcome or diagnostic means to differentiate extensive damage from minor, transient impairment." [Note: This damage resembles acute brain trauma, indicating elevated levels of $S100\beta$, which is a marker of brain damage and blood brain barrier dysfunction]; A. J. Saenz, E. Lee-Lewandrowski, M. J. Wood, T. G. Neilan, A. J. Siegel, J. L. Januzzi, and K. B. Lewandrowski, "Measurement of a Plasma Stroke Biomarker Panel and Cardiac Troponin T in Marathon Runners Before and After the 2005 Boston Marathon," *American Journal of Clinical Pathology* 126, no. 2 (2006): 185–89, "We also

report results of a new plasma biochemical stroke panel in middle-aged nonprofessional athletes before and after the Boston Marathon. The stroke panel consists of 4 biomarkers, S100β, D dimer, BNP, and MMP-9. From the results for various analytes, a software algorithm calculates a stroke index ranging from 1 to 10 with 2 cutoffs: 1.3 or less, low risk; and 5.9 or more, high risk. In terms of individual markers, we observed statistically significant increases in MMP-9 and D dimer levels following competition and no significant change in S100β or BNP levels. The calculated stroke index increased from a mean of 0.97 to 3.5 (P<.001), and 2 subjects had index values above the high-risk cutoff value. We have no clinical or radiologic follow-up data to document the presence or absence of stroke in any of these subjects."

13. H. Schmitt, C. Friebe, S. Schneider, and D. Sabo, "Bone Mineral Density and Degenerative Changes of the Lumbar Spine in Formal Elite Athletes," *International Journal of Sports Medicine* 26, no. 6 (July 2005): 457–63, "The aim of this study was to assess bone mineral density (BMD) and degenerative changes in the lumbar spine in male former elite athletes participating in different track and field disciplines and to determine the influence of body composition and degenerative changes on BMD. One hundred and fifty-nine former male elite athletes (40 throwers, 97 jumpers, 22 endurance athletes) were studied. . . . Throwers had a higher body mass index than jumpers and endurance athletes. Throwers and jumpers had higher BMD (T-LWS) than endurance athletes. Bivariate analysis revealed a negative correlation of BMD (T-score) with age and a positive correlation with BMD and Kellgren score (P<0.05). Even after multiple adjustment for confounders lumbar spine BMD is significantly higher in throwers, pole vaulters, and long- and triple jumpers than in marathon athletes."

14. A. Srivastava, and N. Kreiger, "Relation of Physical Activity to Risk of Testicular Cancer," *American Journal of Epidemiology* 151, no. 1: 78–87.

Chapter 2

1. CNN news story, June 6, 2005, http://edition.cnn.com/2005/health/06/06/sprint.training.

2. K. A. Burgomaster, S. C. Hughes, G. J. F. Heigenhauser, S. N. Bradwell, and M. J. Gibala, "Six Sessions of Sprint Interval Training Increases Muscle Oxidative Potential and Cycle Endurance Capacity in Humans," *Journal of Applied Physiology* 98, no. 6 (June 1, 2005): 1985–90.

3. E. F. Coyle, "Very Intense Exercise-Training Is Extremely Potent and Time Efficient: A Reminder," ibid., 1983–84.

4. Professor Martin (M. J.) Gibala quoted from a CTV interview, ctv. ca/servlet/articlenews/story/ctvnews/1117489599756_13/?hub=health.

5. M. J. Gibala, J. P. Little, M. van Essen, G. P. Wilkin, K. A. Burgomaster, A. Safdar, S. Raha, and M. A. Tarnopolsky, "Short-Term Sprint Interval Versus Traditional Endurance Training: Similar Initial Adaptations in Human Skeletal Muscle and Exercise Performance," *Journal of Physiology* 575 (2006): 901–11.

6. Professor Martin (M. J.) Gibala quoted from a telegraph.co.uk article, telegraph.co.uk/news/main.jhtml?xml=/news/2005/06/05/nfit05.xml.

7. Kenneth Cooper, *The New Aerobics* (New York: Bantam Books, 1970), 17.

8. Ibid., 18.

9. J. G. Salway, *Metabolism at a Glance*, Chapter 26: "Glycogenolysis in Skeletal Muscle," "In the liver glycogenolysis is stimulated by both glucagon and adrenaline, whereas in muscle only adrenaline is effective. In a crisis, when mobilization of glycogen is stimulated by adrenaline, the response must happen immediately. This occurs through the remarkable amplification cascade . . . in which cyclic AMP [adenosine monophosphate] plays an important role. In this way small nanomolar concentrations of adrenaline can rapidly mobilize a vast number of glucose residues for use as respiratory fuel"; Ibid., "Glycogenolysis in muscle is stimulated in muscle via the amplification cascade . . . phosphorylase produces glucose-1-phosphate, which is converted into glucose-6-phosphate. Because muscle lacks glucose-6-phosphate, glucose-6-phosophate is totally committed to glycolysis for ATP production. Also, since muscle hexokinase has a very low KM [or rate of metabolism] for glucose, it has a very high affinity for glucose and will readily phosphorylate to 10% of glucose units liberated from glycogen by the debranching enzyme as free glucose, thus ensuring its use by glycolysis. It should be remembered that adrenaline increases the cyclic AMP concentration, which not only stimulates glycogenolysis, but in muscle also stimulates glycolysis"; Ibid., "The glycogenolysis cascade shows how

the original signal provided by a single molecule of adrenaline is amplified during the course of a cascade of reactions, which activate a large number of phosphorylase molecules, ensuring the rapid mobilization of glycogen as follows:

"1. A molecule of adrenaline stimulates adeno cyclades to form several molecules of cyclic AMP. Each individual ?? of cyclic AMP dissociates an inactive tetrimer to two free catically active units of cyclic AMP dependent protein kinase (also known as protein kinase-A). This gives a relatively modest amplification factor of 2.

"2. Each active molecule of cyclic AMP dependent protein kinase phosphorylates and activates several molecules of phorylase kinase [so, now we're three steps down]. At this point reciprocal regulation of glycogen synthesis and breakdown occurs. First let us continue with glycogenolysis before concluding with an inactivation of glycogen synthesis. One molecule of phosphorylase kinase phosphorylates several inactive molecules of phosphorylase-B, to give the active form of phosphorylase-A, so glycogen breakdown can now proceed."

10. Ibid., "During exercise periods of stress or starvation the triacylglycerol reserves in adipose tissue are mobilized as fatty acids for oxidation as a restoratory fuel. This is analogous to the mobilization of glycogen as glucose units. It occurs under similar circumstances and is under similar hormonal control. Fatty acids are a very important energy substrate in muscle and also in liver where they are metabolized to the ketone bodies. Because fatty acids are hydrophobic, they are transported in the blood bound to albumin (a protein that is soluble in liquid). They can serve most cells as a restoratory fuel with the notable exceptions of the brain and red blood cells, which lack the enzymes for fatty acid oxidation. Regulation of the utilization of fatty acids appears to be at four levels:

"1. Glycolysis of triacylglycerol to form free fatty acids.

"2. Reesterification of fatty acids, or alternatively, their mobilization from adipose tissue.

"3. The transport of the Acetyl-CoA esters into the mitochondria.

"4. Availability of FAD and NADH for Beta oxidation.

"Glycolysis & Adipose Tissue"

"Glycolysis and adipose tissue are controlled by hormone-sensitive lipase. Other synonyms for this enzyme are triacylglycerol lipase and mobilizing lipase. This enzyme hydrolyzes triacylglycerol to monoacylglycerol, which is in turn hydrolyzed to monoacylglycerol lipase. For example, tripolitan is converted to three molecules of polytate and glycerol. Glycolysis is stimulated by adrenaline during exercise, by glucagon during fasting, and by adenacoritcotrophic hormone during starvation. The mechanism involves cyclic AMP dependent protein kinase that both stimulates hormone-sensitive lipase and inhibits Acetyl-CoA carboxylase (ACC). Furthermore, as a long term adaptation to prolonged starvation, cortisol stimulates hormone-sensitive lipase as well. Conversely, in the well-fed state, hormone-sensitive lipase is inhibited by insulin."

11. S. B. Stromme, et al., "Assessment of Maximal Aerobic Power in Specifically Trained Athletes," *Journal of Applied Physiology* 42 (Issue 6) (1977), 833–37. This study measured VO_2 max in athletes and found VO_2 max improvements to be expressed only in their specific sports. For example, elite cross-country skiers showed a ski VO_2 max that was significantly higher than VO_2 max measured during running. This argues that VO_2 max is a sport-specific muscle adaptation (economy of effort) as opposed to a central CV adaptation.; J. R. Magel, et al., "Specificity of Swim Training on Maximal Oxygen Uptake," *Journal of Applied Physiology* 38 (Issue 1) (1975), 151–55. In this study, swim-interval training was performed with young male subjects one hour per day, three days per week, for ten weeks. Swim-trained subjects increased their swim VO_2 max significantly, but there was no significant change in run VO_2 max. This is the same conclusion reached in the Stromme study.

12. B. Saltin, et al., "The Nature of the Training Response: Peripheral and Central Adaptations of One-Legged Exercise," *Acta Physiologica Scandinavica* 96, no. 3 (March 1976): 289–305.

CHAPTER 3

1. H. S. Milner-Brown, R. B. Stein, and R. Yemm, "The Orderly Recruitment of Human Motor Units During Voluntary Isometric Contractions," *Journal of Physiology* 230, no. 2 (April 1973): 359–70; H. S. Milner-Brown, R. B. Stein, and R. Yemm, "Changes in Firing Rate of Human Motor Units

During Linearly Changing Voluntary Contractions," *Journal of Physiology* 230, no. 2 (April 1973): 371–90. See also *Journal of Neurophysiology* 55, no. 5 (May 1986): 1017–29, and *Journal of Neurophysiology* 57, no. 1 (January 1987): 311–24.

2. K. J. Ostrowski, G. J. Wilson, R. Weatherby, P. W. Murphy, and A. D. Lyttle, "The Effect of Weight Training Volume on Hormonal Output and Muscular Size and Function," *Journal of Strength and Conditioning Research* 11, no. 3 (August 1997): 148–54.

3. R.N. Carpinelli and R. M. Otto, "Strength Training: Single Versus Multiple Sets," *Sports Medicine* 26, no. 2 (1998): 73–84.

4. W. Wescott, K. Greenberger, and D. Milius, "Strength Training Research: Sets and Repetitions," *Scholastic Coach* 58 (1989): 98–100.

5. D. Starkey, M. Welsch, and M. Pollock, "Equivalent Improvement in Strength Following High Intensity, Low and High Volume Training," (Paper presented at the annual meeting of the American College of Sports Medicine, Indianapolis, IN, June 2, 1994).

6. D. Starkey, M. Pollock, Y. Ishida, M. A. Welsch, W. Brechue, J. E. Graves, and M. S. Feigenbaum, "Effect of Resistance Training Volume on Strength and Muscle Thickness," *Medicine and Science in Sports and Exercise* 28, no. 10 (October 1996): 1311–20.

7. P. M. Clarkson and K. Nosaka, "Muscle Function After Exercise-Induced Muscle Damage and Rapid Adaptation," *Medicine and Science in Sports and Exercise* 24, no. 5 (1992): 512–20; C. L. Golden and G. A. Dudley, "Strength After Bouts of Eccentric or Concentric Actions," *Medicine and Science in Sports and Exercise* 24, no. 8 (1992) 926–33; P. M. Clarkson and I. Tremblay, "Exercise-Induced Muscle Damage, Repair and Adaptation in Humans," *Journal of Applied Physiology* 65, no. 1 (1998): 1–6; J. N. Howell, G. Chleboun, and R. Conaster, "Muscle Stiffness, Strength Loss, Swelling and Soreness Following Exercise-Induced Injury to Humans," *Journal of Physiology* 464 (1993): 183–96; D. K. Mishra, J. Friden et al., "Anti-Inflammatory Medication After Muscle Injury," *Journal of Bone and Joint Surgery* 77-A, no. 10 (August 1995): 1510–19; L. L. Smith, "Acute Inflammation: The Underlying Mechanism in Delayed Onset Muscle Soreness?" *Medicine and Science in Sports and Exercise* 23, no. 5 (1991): 542–51; P. M. Tiidus and D. C. Ianuzzo, "Effects of Intensity and Duration of Muscular Exercise on Delayed Soreness and

Serum Enzyme Activities," *Medicine and Science in Sports and Exercise* 15, no. 6 (1983): 461–65.

8. P. M. Clarkson and I. Tremblay, "Exercise-Induced Muscle Damage, Repair and Adaptation in Humans," *Journal of Applied Physiology* 65, no. 1 (1998): 1–6; L. L. Smith, "Acute Inflammation: The Underlying Mechanism in Delayed Onset Muscle Soreness?" *Medicine and Science in Sports and Exercise* 23, no. 5 (1991): 542–51.

9. P. M. Clarkson and K. Nosaka, "Muscle Function After Exercise-Induced Muscle Damage and Rapid Adaptation," *Medicine and Science in Sports and Exercise* 24, no. 5 (1992): 512–20; P. M. Tiidus and D. C. Ianuzzo, "Effects of Intensity and Duration of Muscular Exercise on Delayed Soreness and Serum Enzyme Activities," *Medicine and Science in Sports and Exercise* 15, no. 6 (1983): 461–65.

10. P. M. Clarkson and K. Nosaka, "Muscle Function After Exercise-Induced Muscle Damage and Rapid Adaptation," *Medicine and Science in Sports and Exercise* 24, no. 5 (1992): 512–20; D. A. Jones, J. M. Newham, et al., "Experimental Human Muscle Damage: Morphological Changes in Relation to Other Indices of Damage," *Journal of Physiology* 375 (1986) : 435–48; L. L. Smith, "Acute Inflammation: The Underlying Mechanism in Delayed Onset Muscle Soreness?" *Medicine and Science in Sports and Exercise* 23, no. 5 (1991): 542–51.

11. J. Friden et al., "Myofibrillar Damage Following Intense Eccentric Exercise in Man," *International Journal of Sports Medicine* 24, no. 3 (1983): 170–76; D. A. Jones, J. M. Newham et al., "Experimental Human Muscle Damage: Morphological Changes in Relation to Other Indices of Damage," *Journal of Physiology* 375 (1986): 435–48; D. J. Newman and D. A. Jones, "Repeated High-Force Eccentric Exercise: Effects on Muscle Pain and Damage," *Journal of Applied Physiology* 4, no. 63 (1987): 1381–86; L. L. Smith, "Acute Inflammation: The Underlying Mechanism in Delayed Onset Muscle Soreness?" *Medicine and Science in Sports and Exercise* 23, no. 5 (1991): 542–51; P. M. Tiidus and D. C. Ianuzzo, "Effects of Intensity and Duration of Muscular Exercise on Delayed Soreness and Serum Enzyme Activities," *Medicine and Science in Sports and Exercise* 15, no. 6 (1983): 461–65.

12. J. Friden, et al., "Myofibrillar Damage Following Intense Eccentric Exercise in Man," *International Journal of Sports Medicine* 24, no. 3 (1983): 170–76; D. A. Jones, J. M. Newham, et al., "Experimental Human Muscle

Damage: Morphological Changes in Relation to Other Indices of Damage," *Journal of Physiology* 375 (1986): 435–48; P. M. Clarkson and I. Tremblay, "Exercise-Induced Muscle Damage, Repair and Adaptation in Humans," *Journal of Applied Physiology* 65, no.1 (1998): 1–6; C. L. Golden and G. A. Dudley, "Strength After Bouts of Eccentric or Concentric Actions," *Medicine and Science in Sports and Exercise* 24, no. 8 (1992) 926–33; J. N. Howell, G. Chleboun, and R. Conaster, "Muscle Stiffness, Strength Loss, Swelling and Soreness Following Exercise-Induced Injury to Humans," *Journal of Physiology* 464 (1993): 183–96; D. A. Jones, J. M. Newham, et al., "Experimental Human Muscle Damage: Morphological Changes in Relation to Other Indices of Damage," *Journal of Physiology* 375 (1986): 435–48; D. K. Mishra, J. Friden, et al., "Anti-Inflammatory Medication After Muscle Injury," *Journal of Bone and Joint Surgery* 77-A, no. 10 (August 1995): 1510–19; L. L. Smith, "Acute Inflammation: The Underlying Mechanism in Delayed Onset Muscle Soreness?" *Medicine and Science in Sports and Exercise* 23, no. 5 (1991): 542–51; P. M. Tiidus and D. C. Ianuzzo, "Effects of Intensity and Duration of Muscular Exercise on Delayed Soreness and Serum Enzyme Activities," *Medicine and Science in Sports and Exercise* 15, no. 6 (1983): 461–65.

13. P. M. Clarkson and K. Nosaka, "Muscle Function After Exercise-Induced Muscle Damage and Rapid Adaptation," *Medicine and Science in Sports and Exercise* 24, no. 5 (1992): 512–20; D. A. Jones, J. M. Newham, et al., "Experimental Human Muscle Damage: Morphological Changes in Relation to Other Indices of Damage," *Journal of Physiology* 375 (1986): 435–48; D. K. Mishra, J. Friden, et al., "Anti-Inflammatory Medication After Muscle Injury," *Journal of Bone and Joint Surgery* 77-A, no. 10 (August 1995): 1510–19; L. L. Smith, "Acute Inflammation: The Underlying Mechanism in Delayed Onset Muscle Soreness?" *Medicine and Science in Sports and Exercise* 23, no. 5 (1991): 542–51.

14. C. L. Golden and G. A. Dudley, "Strength After Bouts of Eccentric or Concentric Actions," *Medicine and Science in Sports and Exercise* 24, no. 8 (1992) 926–33; D. K. Mishra, J. Friden, et al., "Anti-Inflammatory Medication After Muscle Injury," *Journal of Bone and Joint Surgery* 77-A, no. 10 (August 1995): 1510–19; L. L. Smith, "Acute Inflammation: The Underlying Mechanism in Delayed Onset Muscle Soreness?" *Medicine and Science in Sports and Exercise* 23, no. 5 (1991): 542–51.

15. P. M. Clarkson and I. Tremblay, "Exercise-Induced Muscle Damage, Repair and Adaptation in Humans," *Journal of Applied Physiology* 65, no. 1 (1998): 1–6; C. L. Golden and G. A. Dudley, "Strength After Bouts of Eccentric or Concentric Actions," *Medicine and Science in Sports and Exercise* 24, no. 8 (1992) 926–33; J. N. Howell, G. Chleboun, and R. Conaster, "Muscle Stiffness, Strength Loss, Swelling and Soreness Following Exercise-Induced Injury to Humans," *Journal of Physiology* 464 (1993): 183–96; P. M. Tiidus and D. C. Ianuzzo, "Effects of Intensity and Duration of Muscular Exercise on Delayed Soreness and Serum Enzyme Activities," *Medicine and Science in Sports and Exercise* 15, no. 6 (1983): 461–65.

16. P. M. Clarkson and K. Nosaka, "Muscle Function After Exercise-Induced Muscle Damage and Rapid Adaptation," *Medicine and Science in Sports and Exercise* 24, no.5 (1992): 512–20; P. M. Clarkson and I. Tremblay, "Exercise-Induced Muscle Damage, Repair and Adaptation in Humans," *Journal of Applied Physiology* 65, no. 1 (1998): 1–6; J. Friden, et al. "Myofibrillar Damage Following Intense Eccentric Exercise in Man," *International Journal of Sports Medicine* 24, no. 3 (1983): 170–76; C. L. Golden and G. A. Dudley, "Strength After Bouts of Eccentric or Concentric Actions," *Medicine and Science in Sports and Exercise* 24, no. 8 (1992): 926–33; J. N. Howell, G. Chleboun, and R. Conaster, "Muscle Stiffness, Strength Loss, Swelling and Soreness Following Exercise-Induced Injury to Humans," *Journal of Physiology* 464 (1993): 183–96; D. A. Jones, J. M. Newham, et al., "Experimental Human Muscle Damage: Morphological Changes in Relation to Other Indices of Damage," *Journal of Physiology* 375 (1986): 435–48; D. K. Mishra, J. Friden, et al., "Anti-Inflammatory Medication After Muscle Injury," *Journal of Bone and Joint Surgery* 77-A, no. 10 (August 1995): 1510–19; D. J. Newman and D. A. Jones, "Repeated High-Force Eccentric Exercise: Effects on Muscle Pain and Damage," *Journal of Applied Physiology* 4, no. 63 (1987): 1381–86; L. L. Smith, "Acute Inflammation: The Underlying Mechanism in Delayed Onset Muscle Soreness?" *Medicine and Science in Sports and Exercise* 23, no. 5 (1991): 542–51; P. M. Tiidus and D. C. Ianuzzo, "Effects of Intensity and Duration of Muscular Exercise on Delayed Soreness and Serum Enzyme Activities," *Medicine and Science in Sports and Exercise* 15, no. 6 (1983): 461–65.

17. D. R. Taafe, C. Duret, S. Wheeler, and R. Marcus, "Once-Weekly Resistance Exercise Improves Muscle Strength and Neuromuscular

Performance in Older Adults," *Journal of the American Geriatric Society* 47, no. 10 (October 1999): 1208–14; J. R. McLester, P. Bishop, and M. E. Guilliams, "Comparison of 1 Day and 3 Days per Week of Equal-Volume Resistance Training in Experienced Subjects," *Journal of Strength and Conditioning Research* 14 (2000): 273–81. (In this study subjects who had an average training history of 5.7 years were put on a whole-body training program, consisting of nine exercises performed either one or three times per week. After the study, a post-test conducted on eight out of the nine strength measures indicated that there was no statistical difference between the two groups, which led the researchers to conclude that training once per week delivered the same results as training three times per week.)

18. B. J. Wilson and J. M. Willardson, "A Comparison of Once Versus Twice per Week Training on Leg Press Strength in Women," *Journal of Sports Medicine and Physical Fitness* 47, no.1 (March 2007): 13–17. Conclusion: "These results indicate that performing a single set of leg press once or twice per week results in statistically similar strength gains in untrained women."

19. J. E. Graves, et al., "Effect of Reduced Training Frequency on Muscular Strength," *International Journal of Sports Medicine* 9, no. 5 (1998): 316–19; C. DeRenne, "Effects of Training Frequency on Strength Maintenance in Pubescent Baseball Players," *Journal of Strength and Conditioning Research* 10, no. 1 (1996): 8–14.

20. D. R. Taaffe, R. Dennis, C. Duert, S. Wheeler, and R. Marcus, "Once-Weekly Resistance Training Improves Muscle Strength and Neuromuscular Performance in Older Adults," *Journal of the American Geriatric Society* 47, no. 10 (October 1999): 1208–14.

CHAPTER 4

1. B. T. Boyer, "A Comparison of the Effects of Three Strength Training Programs on Women," *Journal of Applied Sports Science Research* 4, Issue 5 (1990): 88–94; M. T. Sanders, "A Comparison of Two Methods of Training on the Development of Muscular Strength and Endurance," *Journal of Orthopaedic and Sports Physical Therapy* 1 (1980): 210–13; L. J. Silvester, C. Stiggins, C. McGown, and G. R. Bryce, "The Effect of Variable Resistance

and Free-Weight Training Programs on Strength and Vertical Jump," *NSCA Journal* 3, no. 6 (1982): 30–33.

2. K. Jones, P. Bishop, G. Hunter, and G. Fleisig, "The Effects of Varying Resistance Training Loads on Intermediate and High Velocity Specific Adaptations," *Journal of Strength Conditioning Research* 15 (2001): 349–56.

3. J. G. Hay, J. G. Andrews, and C. L. Vaughan, "Effects of Lifting Rate on Elbow Torques Exerted During Arm Curl Exercises," *Medicine and Science in Sports and Exercise* 15, no. 1 (1983): 63–71.

4. W. L. Wescott, et al., "Effects of Regular and Slow Speed Resistance Training on Muscle Strength," *Journal of Sports Medicine and Physical Fitness* 41, no. 2 (2001): 154–58.

5. D. H. Kuland, *The Injured Athlete* (Philadelphia: J. B. Lippincott, 1982); S. Hall, "Effect of Lifting Speed on Forces and Torque Exerted on the Lumbar Spine," *Medicine and Science in Sports and Exercise* 17, no. 4 (1985): 440–44; P. T. Kotani, N. Ichikawa, W. Wakabayaski, T. Yoshii, and M. Koshimuni, "Studies of Spondylolysis Found Among Weightlifters," *British Journal of Sports Medicine* 6 (1971): 4–8; and M. Duda, "Elite Lifters at Risk of Spondylolysis," *Physician and Sports Medine* 5, no. 9 (1977): 61–67.

6. R. Cooke, "The Inhibition of Rabbit Skeletal Muscle Contraction by Hydrogen Ions and Phosphate," *Journal of Physiology* 395 (1988): 77–97; D. G. Stephenson, G. D. Lamb, and G. M. Stephenson, "Events of the Excitation-Contraction-Relaxation Cycle in Fast- and Slow-Twitch Mammalian Muscle Fibres Relevant to Muscle Fatigue," *Acta Physiologica Scandinavica* 162 (1998): 229–45; D. J. Chasiotis, "ATP Utilization and Force During Intermittent and Continuous Muscle Contractions," *Journal of Applied Physiology* 63 (1987): 167–74; M. C. Hogan, "Contraction Duration Affects Metabolic Energy Cost and Fatigue in Skeletal Muscle," *American Journal of Physiology—Endocrinology and Metabolism* 274 (1998): E397–E402; L. Spriet, "ATP Utilization and Provision in Fast-Twitch Skeletal Muscle During Tetanic Contractions," *American Journal of Physiology—Endocrinology and Metabolism* 257 (1989): E595–E605; and H. Barcrof, "The Blood Flow Through Muscle During Sustained Contraction," *Journal of Physiology* 97 (1939): 17–31.

7. G. E. Plopper, "Convergence of Integrin and Growth Factor Receptor Signaling Pathways Within the Focal Adhesion Complex," *Molecular Biology of the Cell* 6 (1995): 1349–65; H. Sackin, "Mechanosensitive

Channels," *Annual Review of Physiology* 57 (1995): 333–53; T. A. Hornberger, "Mechanical Stimuli Regulate Rapamycin-Sensitive Signaling by a Phosphoinositide 3-Kinase-, Protein Kinase B- and Growth Factor-Independent Mechanism," *Biochemistry Journal* 380 (2004): 795–804; and J. S. Kim et al., "Impact of Resistance Loading on Myostatin Expression and Cell Cycle Regulation in Young and Older Men and Women," *American Journal of Physiology—Endocrinology and Metabolism* 288, no. 6 (June 2005): E1110–E1119.

8. K. Hakkinen and A. Pakarinen, "Acute Hormonal Responses to Two Different Fatiguing Heavy-Resistance Protocols in Male Athletes," *Journal of Applied Physiology* 74, no. 2 (February 1993): 882–87. (This study compared a series of single-rep max lifts—twenty sets at 1 rep max (RM) versus 70 percent 1 RM performed until fatigue. Only the 70 percent protocol with inroad/fatigue produced increases in free testosterone and GH and correlated with accumulation of blood lactate in the 70 percent fatiguing protocol. This article also supports accumulated by-products of fatigue) J. L. Rivero et al., "Contribution of Exercise Intensity and Duration to Training-Linked Myosin Transitions in Thoroughbreds," *Equine Veterinary Journal Supplements* 36 (August 2006): 311–15, "The short-term training-induced up-regulation of HMC IIA and down-regulation of MHC IIX in thoroughbreds are more dependent on intensity than duration of exercise." This article correlates intensity by lactate levels and thus can also support accumulated by-products of fatigue; J. L. Rivero, et al. "Effects of Intensity and Duration of Exercise on Muscular Responses to Training of Thoroughbred Racehorses," *Journal of Applied Physiology* 102, no. 5 (May 2007): 1871–82. Same study as preceding. (Note: Doug McGuff's literature police strike again. Editorial/peer review is supposed to make certain that authors don't double-dip on their publishing and that submitted articles represent new knowledge not presented elsewhere. The *Journal of Applied Physiology* is a big-name journal that should not have let this slip under the radar.); and M. Izguierdo, J. Ibañez, et al., "Differential Effects of Strength Training Leading to Failure Versus Not to Failure on Hormonal Responses, Strength, and Muscle Power Gains," *Journal of Applied Physiology* 100, no. 5 (May 2006): 1647–56. This study showed similar strength increases but greater cortisol and less testosterone in failure training than not-to-failure training. However, volume and frequency were not adjusted to compensate

for the higher intensity of failure training. Nevertheless, the advantages of inroad (or positive failure) training can be seen—same strength, less time.

CHAPTER 5

1. K. Koffler, A. Menkes, A. Redmond, et al., "Strength Training Accelerates Gastrointestinal Transit in Middle-Aged and Older Men," *Medicine and Science in Sports and Exercise* 24, no. 4 (1992): 415–19.

2. W. J. Evans and I. Rosenberg, *Biomarkers* (New York: Simon & Schuster, 1992), 44; A. Keys, H. L. Taylor, and F. Grande, "Basal Metabolism and Age of Adult Men," *Metabolism* 22 (1973): 579–87.

3. W. Campbell, M. Crim, C. Young, and W. Evans, "Increased Energy Requirements and Changes in Body Composition with Resistance Training in Older Adults," *American Journal of Clinical Nutrition* 60 (1994): 167–75.

4. B. Hurley, "Does Strength Training Improve Health Status?" *Strength and Conditioning Journal* 16 (1994): 7–13.

5. M. Stone, D. Blessing, R. Byrd, et al., "Physiological Effects of a Short Term Resistive Training Program on Middle-Aged Untrained Men," *National Strength and Conditioning Association Journal* 4 (1982): 16–20; B. Hurley, J. Hagberg, A. Goldberg, et al., "Resistance Training Can Reduce Coronary Risk Factors Without Altering VO_2 Max or Percent Bodyfat," *Medicine and Science in Sports and Exercise* 20 (1988): 150–54.

6. K. A. Harris and R. G. Holly, "Physiological Response to Circuit Weight Training in Borderline Hypertensive Subjects," *Medicine and Science in Sports and Exercise* 19, no. 3 (June 19, 1987): 246–52. This study revealed that resting or exercise blood pressure was not adversely affected and that blood pressure lowered at the end of the study period. In other words, strength training lowered blood pressure without risk of dangerous blood pressure increases during the training period.; E. B. Colliander and P. A. Tesch, "Blood Pressure in Resistance-Trained Athletes," *Canadian Journal of Applied Sports Sciences* 13, no. 1 (March 1988): 31–34. Conclusion: "Intense long-term strength training, as performed by bodybuilders, does not constitute a potential cardiovascular risk factor."

7. A. Menkes, S. Mazel, A. Redmond, et al., "Strength Training Increases Regional Bone Mineral Density and Bone Remodeling in Middle-Aged and Older Men," *Journal of Applied Physiology* 74 (1993): 2478–84.

8. D. Kerr, et al., "Exercise Effects on Bone Mass in Postmenopausal Women Are Site-Specific and Load-Dependent," *Journal of Bone and Mineral Research* 11, no. 2 (February 1996): 218–25.

9. Manohar Pahjabi, et al., "Spinal Stability and Intersegmental Muscle Forces: A Biomechanical Model," *Spine* 14, no. 2 (1989), 194–200.

10. "Never Too Late to Build Up Your Muscle," *Tufts University Diet and Nutrition Letter* 12 (September 1994): 6–7.

11. L. C. Rail, et al., "The Effect of Progressive Resistance Training in Rheumatoid Arthritis: Increased Strength Without Changes in Energy Balance or Body Composition," *Arthritis Rheum* 39, no. 3 (March 1996): 415–26.

12. B. W. Nelson, E. O'Reilly, M. Miller, M. Hogan, C. E. Kelly, and J. A. Wegner, "The Clinical Effects of Intensive Specific Exercise on Chronic Low Back Pain: A Controlled Study of 895 Consecutive Patients with 1-Year Follow Up," *Orthopedics* 18, no. 10 (October 1995), 971–81.

13. S. Leggett, V. Mooney, L. N. Matheson, B. Nelson, T. Dreisinger, J. Van Zytveld, and L. Vie, "Restorative Exercise for Clinical Low Back Pain (A Prospective Two-Center Study with 1-Year Follow Up)," *Spine* 24, no. 9 (November 1999).

14. S. Risch, N. Nowell, M. Pollock, et al., "Lumbar Strengthening in Chronic Low Back Pain Patients," *Spine* 18 (1993): 232–38.

15. A. Faigenbaum, L. Zaichkowsky, W. Westcott, et al., "Effects of Twice per Week Strength Training Program on Children" (paper presented at the annual meeting of the New England Chapter of American College of Sports Medicine, Boxborough, MA, November 12, 1992).

16. W. Westcott, "Keeping Fit," *Nautilus* 4, no. 2 (1995): 5–7.

17. S. P. Messier and M. E. Dill, "Alterations in Strength and Maximum Oxygen Consumption Consequent to Nautilus Circuit Weight Training," *Research Quarterly for Exercise and Sport* 56, no. 4 (1985): 345–51. Conclusion: "The results of this study suggest that for a training period of short duration, Nautilus circuit weight training appears to be an

equally effective alternative to standard free weight (strength) and aerobic (endurance) training programs for untrained individuals." The authors state that there was a significant increase in VO_2 max in the Nautilus group and add, "There was no significant difference between the Nautilus and Run groups" in VO_2 max; L. Goldberg and K. S. Elliot, "Cardiovascular Changes at Rest and During Mixed Static and Dynamic Exercise After Weight Training," *Journal of Applied Science Research* 2, no. 3 (1988): 42–45. Conclusion: "Traditional, non-circuit weight training for both the athlete and the general population can be viewed as a method of reducing myocardial oxygen demand during usual daily activities. This cardio-protective benefit allows the individual to perform isometric exertion combined with dynamic work with lower cardiac oxygen requirements, and, thus, improvement in cardiovascular efficiency. . . . [C]ardiovascular benefits do occur."

18. K. Meyer, et al. "Hemodynamic Responses During Leg Press Exercise in Patients with Chronic Congestive Heart Failure," *American Journal of Cardiology* 83, no. 11 (June 1999): 1537–43.

19. M. A. Rogers and W. J. Evans, "Changes in Skeletal Muscle with Aging: Effects of Exercise Training," *Exercise and Sport Science Reviews* 21 (1993): 65–102.

20. W. D. Daub, G. P. Knapik, and W. R. Black, "Strength Training Early After Myocardial Infarction," *Journal of Cardiopulmonary Rehabilitation* 16, no. 2 (March 1996): 100–8. This study compared use of aerobic and strength training during a cardiac rehab program. Thirty of forty-two subjects had a complication (arrhythmia, angina, ischemia, hypertension, or hypotension) during aerobic exercise. Only one subject had a complication during strength training, and this was a harmless arrhythmia. This shows that strength training is cardioprotective and most likely enhances coronary artery blood flow; D. W. DeGroot, et al., "Circuit Weight Training in Cardiac Patients: Determining Optimal Workloads for Safety and Energy Expenditure," *Journal of Cardiopulmonary Rehabilitation* 18, no. 2 (March–April 1998): 145–52. Subjects with documented coronary artery disease performed aerobic exercise or circuit weight training. The heart rate and rate pressure product were lower during circuit weight training than at 85 percent treadmill VO_2 max. There was no angina or ST depression (signs of compromised coronary artery blood flow) during circuit weight training; Y.

Beniamini, et al., "High-Intensity Strength Training of Patients Enrolled in an Outpatient Cardiac Rehabilitation Program," *Journal of Cardiopulmonary Rehabilitation* 19, no. 1 (January–February 1999): 8–17. Subjects were randomized to high-intensity training versus flexibility training. The high-intensity training group lost more bodyfat, gained lean tissue, and improved treadmill time. No cardiac ischemia or arrhythmia occurred during the training session. Improvements in flexibility were the same in both groups. Again, all the improvements were realized with none of the risk; M. J. Haykowsky, et al., "Effects of Long Term Resistance Training on Left Ventricular Morphology," *Canadian Journal of Cardiology* 16, no. 1 (January 2000: 35–38. Conclusion: "Contrary to common beliefs, long term resistance training as performed by elite male power-lifters does not alter left ventricular morphology." No adverse effects on the heart were found, even with power lifters.

21. K. Hutchins, *SuperSlow: The Ultimate Exercise Protocol* (Casselberry, FL: Media Support/SuperSlow Systems, 1992).

22. W. Wescott, "Exercise Speed and Strength Development," *American Fitness Quarterly* 13, no. 3:20–21.

23. W. Wescott, et al., "Effects of Regular and Slow Speed Training on Muscle Strength," *Master Trainer* 9, no. 4:14–17.

CHAPTER 6

1. A. L. Goldberg, J. D. Etlinger, D. F. Goldspink, and C. Jablecki, "Mechanism of Work-Induced Hypertrophy of Skeletal Muscle," *Medicine and Science in Sports and Exercise* 7, no. 3 (Fall 1975): 185–98.

2. R. G. McMurray and C. F. Brown, "The Effect of Sleep Loss on High Intensity Exercise and Recovery," *Aviation, Space, and Environmental Medicine* 55, no. 11 (November 1984): 1031–35.

3. D. A. Judelson, et al., "Effect of Hydration State on Strength, Power, and Resistance Exercise Performance," *Medicine and Science in Sports and Exercise* 39, no. 10 (October 2007): 1817–24; Ibid., "Hydration and Muscular Performance: Does Fluid Balance Affect Strength, Power and High-Intensity Endurance?" *Sports Medicine* 37, no. 10 (2007): 907–21; R. W. Kenefick, et al., "Hypohydration Adversely Affects Lactate Threshold in

Endurance Athletes," *Journal of Strength Conditional Research* 16, no. 1 (February 2002): 38–43.

4. C. M. Maresh, et al., "Effect of Hydration State on Testosterone and Cortisol Responses to Training-Intensity Exercise in Collegiate Runners," *International Journal of Sports Medicine* 27, no. 10 (October 2006): 765–70.

CHAPTER 7

1. J. Howell, G. Chlebow, and R. Conaster. "Muscle Stiffness, Strength Loss, Swelling and Soreness Following Exercise-Induced Injury in Humans." *Journal of Physiology* 464 (May 1993): 183–96. (From the somatic dysfunction research laboratory of the college of osteopathic medicine and the department of biological sciences, at Ohio University, Athens.)

2. J. P. Ahtianinen, et al., "Acute Hormonal and Neuromuscular Responses and Recovery to Forced vs. Maximum Repetitions Multiple Resistance Exercises," *International Journal of Sports Medicine* 24, no. 6 (August 2003): 410–18.

3. C. D. Massey, J. Vincent, M. Maneval, M. Moore, and J. T. Johnson, "An Analysis of Full Range of Motion vs. Partial Range of Motion Training in the Development of Strength in Untrained Men," *Journal of Strength Conditional Research* 18, no. 3 (2004): 518–21.

4. K. Hakkinen and P. Komi, "Effect of Different Combined Concentric and Eccentric Muscle Work Regimes on Maximal Strength Development," *Journal of Human Movement Studies* 7 (1981): 33–44; L. Ahlquist, R. Hinkle, L. Webber, A. Ward, and J. Rippe, "The Effect of Four Strength Training Programs on Body Composition in Sedentary Men" (paper presented at the National Meeting of the Canadian Association of Sports Sciences, 1991); L. Ahlquist, A. Ward, and J. Rippe, "The Effectiveness of Different Weight-Training Protocols on Muscle Strength and Muscle Cross-Sectional Area: Body Composition and Various Psychological Parameters" (internal report from the Exercise Physiology and Nutrition Laboratory, University of Massachusetts Medical Center, 1991); R. Hinkle, L. Webber, L. Ahlquist, A. Ward, D. Kelleher, and J. Rippe, "The Effect of Different Strength Protocols on Selected Strength Measures" (paper presented at the National Meeting of the Canadian Association of Sports Sciences, 1991); Ibid.,

"The Effect of Added Eccentric Resistance Training on Selected Strength Measures"; E. Colliander and P. Tesch, "Responses to Eccentric and Concentric Resistance Training in Females and Males," *Acta Physiologica Scandinavica* 141 (1990): 149–56; B. Johnson, et al., "A Comparison of Concentric and Eccentric Muscle Training," *Medicine and Science in Sports and Exercise* 8 (1976): 35–38; J. Mannheimer, "A Comparison of Strength Gain Between Concentric and Eccentric Contractions," *Physical Therapy* 49 (1968): 1201–7; V. Seliger, et al., "Adaptations of Trained Athletes' Energy Expenditure to Repeated Concentric and Eccentric Muscle Actions," *International Physiology* 26 (1968): 227–34; P. Tesch, A. Thornsson, and E. Colliander, "Effects of Eccentric and Concentric Resistance Training on Skeletal Muscle Substrates, Enzyme Activities and Capillary Supply," *Acta Physiologica Scandinavica* 140 (1990): 575–80.

5. D. J. Chasiotis, "ATP Utilization and Force During Intermittent and Continuous Muscle Contractions," *Journal of Applied Physiology* 63 (1987): 167–74; M. C. Hogan, "Contraction Duration Affects Metabolic Energy Cost and Fatigue in Skeletal Muscle," *American Journal of Physiology— Endocrinology and Metabolism* 274 (1998): E397–E402; L. Spriet, "ATP Utilization and Provision in Fast-Twitch Skeletal Muscle During Tetanic Contractions," *American Journal of Physiology—Endocrinology and Metabolism* 257 (1989): E595–E605; H. Barcrof, "The Blood Flow Through Muscle During Sustained Contraction," *Journal of Physiology* 97 (1939): 17–31.

Chapter 8

1. M. C. Thibault, et al., "Inheritance of Human Muscle Enzyme Adaptation to Isokinetic Strength Training," *Human Heredity* 36, no. 6 (1986): 341–47. This study subjected five sets of identical twins to a ten-week strength-training program. Biochemical markers of strength were monitored, and there was a wide range of response among the five twin sets, but responses of the identical twins within each set were . . . well . . . identical.

2. S. J. Lee, "Regulation of Muscle Mass by Myostatin," *Annual Review of Cell and Developmental Biology* 20 (November 2004): 61–86. This is a review

article by Se Jin Lee, the chief discoverer of the myostatin gene, and is applicable to almost any aspect of myostatin discussed in this book.

3. Markus Schuelke, et al., "Myostatin Mutation Associated with Gross Muscle Hypertrophy in a Child," *New England Journal of Medicine* 350 (June 24, 2004): 2682–88. This article announced the discovery of the first documented spontaneous deletion of the myostatin gene; the subject was a German child.

4. S. J. Lee, "Sprinting Without Myostatin: A Genetic Determinant of Athletic Prowess," *Trends Genet* 23, issue 10 (October 2007): 475–77. This article discusses how spontaneous deletion in whippets produces an inordinately muscular racing dog that can't be beat; D. S. Mosher, et al., "A Mutation in the Myostatin Gene Increases Muscle Mass and Enhances Racing Performance in Heterozygote Dogs," *PLoS Genet* 3, no. 5 (May 25, 2007): e79, Epub April 30, 2007; S. Shadun, "Genetics: Run, Whippet Run," *Nature* 447 (May 17, 2007): 275.

5. A. Rebbapragada, et al., "Myostatin Signals Through a Transforming Growth Factor Beta-Like Signaling Pathway to Block Adipogenesis," *Molecular and Cell Biology* 23, no. 20 (October 23, 2003): 7230–42. It not only grows muscle but also makes you ripped.

6. C. E. Stewart and J. Rittweger, "Adaptive Processes in Skeletal Muscle: Molecular Regulators and Genetic Influences," *Journal of Musculoskeletal and Neuronal Interactions* 6, no. 1 (January–March 2006): 73–86. This review article nicely covers other genetic factors that control response to exercise and may in the future allow for customization protocols for individuals.

7. N. Yang, et al, "ACTN3 Genotype Is Associated with Human Elite Athletic Performance," *American Journal of Human Genetics* 73, no. 3 (September 2003): 627–41.

8. Nicholas A. Christakis and James Fowler, "The Spread of Obesity in a Large Social Network over 32 Years," *New England Journal of Medicine* 357, no. 4 (July 26, 2007): 370–79.

9. Ethan Waters, "DNA Is Not Destiny," *Discover* 27, no. 11 (November 2006); and Joanne Downer, "Backgrounder: Epigenetics and Imprinted Genes," hopkinsmedicine.org/press/2002/november/epigenetics.htm.

CHAPTER 9

1. E. J. Fine and R. D. Feinman, "Thermodynamics of Weight Loss Diets," *Nutrition and Metabolism* 1 (2004): 15, nutritionandmetabolism.com/content/1/1/15.

2. J. S. Volek and R. D. Feinman, "Carbohydrate Restriction Improves the Features of Metabolic Syndrome: Metabolic Syndrome May Be Defined by the Response to Carbohydrate Restriction," *Nutrition and Metabolism* 2 (2005): 31, nutritionandmetabolism.com/content/2/1/31; J. S. Volek, et al., "Comparison of Energy-Restricted Very-Low Carbohydrate and Low-Fat Diets on Weight Loss and Body Composition in Overweight Men and Women," *Nutrition and Metabolism* 1 (2004): 13, nutritionandmetabolism.com/content/1/1/13; S. J. Peters and P. J. LeBlanc, "Metabolic Aspects of Low Carbohydrate Diets and Exercise," *Nutrition and Metabolism* 1 (2004): 7, nutritionandmetabolism.com/content/1/1/7; Stephen D. Phinney, "Ketogenic Diets and Physical Performance," *Nutrition and Metabolism* 1 (2004): 2, nutritionandmetabolism.com/content/1/1/2.

3. Ellington Darden, *Living Longer Stronger* (New York: Berkeley Publishing Group, 1995), 112. This calculation is based on the amount of heat energy required to warm ingested chilled water to body-temperature urine, minus a small fudge factor for passive warming.

4. D. L. Ballor, V. L. Katch, M. D. Becque, and C. R. Marks, "Resistance Weight Training During Caloric Restriction Enhances Lean Body Weight Maintenance," *American Journal of Clinical Nutrition* 47 (1988): 19–25.

5. Ethan Waters, "DNA Is Not Destiny," *Discover* 27, no. 11 (November 2006).

6. T. V. Kral and B. J. Rolls, "Energy Density and Portion Size: Their Independent and Combined Effects on Energy Intake," *Physiology and Behavior* 82, no. 1 (August 2004): 131–38.

7. "Muscle Hypertrophy with Large-Scale Weight Loss and Resistance Training," *American Journal of Clinical Nutrition* 58 (1993): 561–65.

CHAPTER 10

1. D. Schmidtbleicher, "An Interview on Strength Training for Children," *National Strength and Conditioning Association Bulletin* 9, no. 12 (1988): 42a–42b.

2. K. A. Ericsson, et al., "The Making of an Expert," *Harvard Business Review* 85, (July–August, 2007): 114–21, 193.

3. K. A. Ericsson, R. Krampe, and T. H. Tesch-Romer, "The Role of Deliberate Practice in the Acquisition of Expert Performance," *Psychological Review* 100, no. 3 (1993): 379–84.

4. S. B. Thacker, J. Gilchrist, D. F. Stroup, and C. Dexter Kimsey Jr., "The Impact of Stretching on Sports Injury Risk: A Systematic Review of the Literature," *Medicine and Science in Sports and Exercise* 36, no. 3 (March 2004): 371–78.

5. D. Lally, "New Study Links Stretching with Higher Injury Rates," *Running Research News* 10, no. 3 (1994): 5–6.

6. R. D. Herbert and M. Gabriel, "Effects of Stretching Before and After Exercising on Muscle Soreness and Risk of Injury: Systematic Review," *British Medical Journal* 325 (August 31, 2002): 468.

7. R. P. Pope, R. D. Herbert, J. D. Kirwan, et al., "A Randomized Trial of Preexercise Stretching for Prevention of Lower-Limb Injury," *Medicine and Science in Sports and Exercise* 32, no. 2 (February 2000): 271–77.

8. E. Witvrouw, et al., "The Role of Stretching in Tendon Injuries," *British Journal of Sports Medicine* 41 (January 29, 2007): 224–26.

9. A. G. Nelson, J. B. Winchester, and J. Kokkonen, "A Single Thirty Second Stretch Is Sufficient to Inhibit Maximal Voluntary Strength," *Medicine and Science in Sports and Exercise* 38, Suppl. no. 5 (May 2006): S294.

10. SafeKidsUSA, usa.safekids.org/tier3_cd.cfm?folder_id=540&content_item _id=1211.

CHAPTER 11

1. J. R. Meuleman, et al., "Exercise Training in the Debilitated Aged: Strength and Functional Outcomes," *Archives of Physical Medicine and Rehabilitation* 81, no. 3 (March 2000): 312–18. Fifty-eight elderly subjects with at least

one impairment in activities of daily life completed an eight-week strength-training program. Strength increased an average of 32.8 percent, with the most debilitated showing the greatest improvement. The article states: "This group of debilitated elderly patients effectively performed resistance training and increased their strength, with the most impaired gaining the most function."

2. R. A. Fielding, "Effects of Exercise Training in the Elderly: Impact of Progressive-Resistance Training on Skeletal Muscle and Whole-Body Protein Metabolism," *Proceedings of the Nutrition Society* 54, no. 3 (November 1995): 665–75. This review article states: "The overwhelming evidence presented in the present review suggests that loss of muscle strength and function observed with advancing age is reversible even in the frail elderly. Exercise programs designed to improve muscle strength are recommended for older individuals as an effective countermeasure to the sarcopenia of old age."

3. W. Frontera, C. Meredith, K. O'Reilly, H. Knuttgen, and W. J. Evans, "Strength Conditioning in Older Men: Skeletal Muscle Hypertrophy and Improved Function," *Journal of Applied Physiology* 64, no. 3 (1988): 1038–44; M. Nelson, M. Fiatarone, C. Morganti, I. Trice, R. Greenberg, and W. J. Evans, "Effects of High-Intensity Strength Training on Multiple Risk Factors for Osteoporotic Fractures," *Journal of the American Medical Association* 272, no. 24 (1994): 1909–14; M. Fiatarone, E. O'Neill, N. Ryan, K. Clements, G. Solares, M. Nelson, S. Roberts, J. Kehayias, L Lipsitz, and W. J. Evans, "Exercise Training and Nutritional Supplementation for Physical Frailty in Very Elderly People," *New England Journal of Medicine* 330, no. 25 (1994): 1769–75.

4. P. A. Ades, et al., "Weight Training Improves Walking Endurance in Healthy Elderly Persons," *Annals of Internal Medicine* 124, no. 6 (March 15, 1996): 568–72. Twenty-four subjects sixty-five to seventy-nine years old underwent a three-month weight-training program. Participants increased their walking endurance by 38 percent. There was no change in peak aerobic capacity to account for the improvement. The article states: "Resistance training for 3 months improves both leg strength and walking endurance in healthy, community dwelling elderly persons. This finding is relevant to older persons at risk for disability, because walking endurance and leg strength are important components of physical functioning."

5. W. J. Evans, "Reversing Sarcopenia: How Weight Training Can Build Strength and Vitality," *Geriatrics* 51, no. 5 (May 1996): 46–47, 51–53, "Progressive resistance exercises can produce substantial increases in strength and muscle size, even in the oldest old. For many older patients, resistance training represents the safest, least expensive means to lose body fat, decrease blood pressure, improve glucose tolerance, and maintain long-term independence."

6. W. Campbell, M. Crim, V. Young, and W. J. Evans, "Increased Energy Requirements and Changes in Body Composition with Resistance Training in Older Adults," *American Journal of Clinical Nutrition* 60 (1994): 167–75; R. Pratley, B. Nicklas, M. Rubin, J. Miller, A. Smith, M. Smith, B. Hurley, and A. Goldberg, "Strength Training Increases Resting Metabolic Rate and Norepinephrine Levels in Healthy 50 to 65 Year-Old Men," *Journal of Applied Physiology* 767 (1994): 133–37.

7. K. Harris and R. Holy, "Physiological Response to Circuit Weight Training in Borderline Hypertensive Subjects," *Medicine and Science in Sports and Exercise* 10 (1987): 246–52.

8. M. Stone, D. Blessing, R. Byrd, J. Tew, and D. Boatwright, "Physiological Effects of a Short Term Resistive Training Program on Middle-Aged Untrained Men," *National Strength and Conditioning Association Journal* 4 (1982): 16–20.

9. K. Koffler, A. Menkes, A. Redmond, W. Whitehead, R. Pratley, and B. Hurley, "Strength Training Accelerates Gastrointestinal Transit in Middle-Aged and Older Men," *Medicine and Science in Sports and Exercise* 24 (1992): 415–19.

10. B. Hurley, "Does Strength Training Improve Health Status?" *Strength and Conditioning Journal* 16 (1994): 7–13.

11. S. Risch, N. Nowell, M. Pollock, E. Risch, H. Langer, M. Fulton, J. Graves, and S. Leggett, "Lumbar Strengthening in Chronic Low Back Pain Patients," *Spine* 18 (1993): 232–38.

12. A. Menkes, S. Mazel, R. Redmond, K. Koffler, C. Libanati, C. Gundberg, T. Zizic, J. Hagberg, R. Pratley, and B. Hurley, "Strength Training Increases Regional Bone Mineral Density and Bone Remodeling in Middle-Aged and Older Men," *Journal of Applied Physiology* 74 (1993): 2478–84.

13. See Chap. 5, n. 10.

14. N. Singh, K. Clements, and M. Fiatarone, "A Randomized Controlled Trial of Progressive Resistance Training in Depressed Elders," *Journal of Gerontology* 52A, no. 1 (1997): M27–M35.

15. K. Stewart, M. Mason, and M. Kelemen, "Three-Year Participation in Circuit Weight Training Improves Muscular Strength and Self-Efficacy in Cardiac Patients," *Journal of Cardiopulmonary Rehabilitation* 8 (1998): 292–96.

16. The summary of this study has been published at seniorfitness.net/strength .htm.

17. S. Melov, M. A. Tarnopolsky, K. Beckman, K. Felkey, and A. Hubbard, "Resistance Exercise Reverses Aging in Human Skeletal Muscle," plosone. org/article/info:doi%2f10.1371%2fjournal.pone.0000465.

Index

About the Authors

Doug McGuff, M.D., became interested in exercise at the age of fifteen when he first read Arthur Jones's *Nautilus Training Bulletin* (No. 2). His interest in exercise and biology led him into a career in medicine. In 1989, he graduated from the University of Texas Medical School at San Antonio and went on to train in emergency medicine at the University of Arkansas for Medical Sciences at Little Rock, where he served as chief resident. From there, he served as faculty in the Wright State University Emergency Medicine Residency and was a staff emergency physician at Wright-Patterson AFB Hospital.

Throughout his career, Dr. McGuff has maintained his interest in high-intensity exercise. He realized a lifelong dream when he opened Ultimate Exercise in November 1997 (ultimate-exercise.com). Over the past eleven years, he and his instructors have continued to explore the limits of exercise through their personal training clients at Ultimate Exercise.

In addition to his work at Ultimate Exercise, Dr. McGuff is a partner with Blue Ridge Emergency Physicians, P.A. He lives in Seneca, South Carolina, with his wife of twenty-five years and their children, Eric and Madeline.

John Little is considered "one of the top fitness researchers in North America" (*Ironman* magazine). He first learned of the principles of correct exercise from bodybuilding pioneer Mike Mentzer, when John was eighteen years old. Mentzer encouraged him to continue with his research, which resulted in Little's creation of the Max Contraction training method (maxcontraction.com). Little has authored twelve books on exercise and an additional thirty-eight books on philosophy (Eastern and Western), history, and martial arts. A graduate of McMaster University, Hamilton, with a degree in philosophy, Little has been published in every major fitness and martial arts magazine in North America. Throughout his career, he has worked alongside the biggest names in the industry, including Arnold Schwarzenegger, Steve Reeves, Lou Ferrigno, and Jackie Chan, as well as Mike Mentzer. He is also an award-winning documentary filmmaker, having produced and directed films for both independent companies and major studios such as Warner Bros.

In 2004, Little and his wife, Terri, opened Nautilus North Strength & Fitness Centre, where they continue to conduct studies on exercise and share the data with their personal training clients. Nautilus North has supervised in excess of sixty thousand one-on-one workout sessions. Little has continued to perpetuate the teachings and legacy of Mike Mentzer, carrying on Mentzer's "Heavy Duty" column in *Ironman* magazine since Mentzer's passing in 2001. He lives in Bracebridge, Ontario, with his wife of twenty years and their children, Riley, Taylor, Brandon, and Benjamin.

If you would like more information on the science of productive exercise, the authors welcome you to visit Body by Science online at bodyby science.net.